Honestly, MAN

Why masculinity feels confusing, shame doesn't help and what to do about it

ANDREW PAIN

Honestly, Man

Paperback ISBN 978-1-917490-44-3

eISBN 978-1-917490-45-0

Published in 2026 by Right Book Press

Printed in the UK in June 2026

Manufactured by
Sue Richardson Associates Ltd.
Studio 6,
9, Marsh Street
Bristol
BS1 4AA

info@therightbookcompany.com

A CIP record of this book is available from the British Library.

Contents

Introduction

I'm worried. I've always been a worrier and, as a father of five, worrying is part of the job, right? But seriously, I'm worried, and I'm guessing that since you picked this book up, you might be too.

Another day, another stabbing. The vast majority of knife crime victims (and perpetrators) are boys or men, and I can't help but wonder, what if that happened to one of my three boys? Statistically it's unlikely, given their privileges as children (stable family home, middle-class neighbourhood), but it could and does happen.

Another day, and according to annual data from the UK Office for National Statistics (ONS 2024b), 12 men in England and Wales will have died today by suicide, leaving shattered families, devastated friends and fractured communities. I have a dad, I have sons, brothers-in-law and plenty of male friends. It breaks my heart how frequently I hear from a mate or peer that they've attended the funeral of a guy who died by suicide. What if I lost one of my own family members that way?

Another day, and social media spins the toxic masculinity and 'kill all men' narratives on the one hand, while spreading misogynistic rubbish on the other. At the same time, social inequality and the struggle to make ends meet are worsening issues for most people, creating a bleak and polarised picture. It's not surprising that the number of disaffected, resentful men is increasing. I don't want to be part of a divided society. I doubt you want that either.

We could just put our heads in the sand and pretend it's not happening. Even if we wanted to make a difference, when the issues are so all-consuming and complex, where would we start? It may feel easier to blame people like controversial influencer Andrew Tate, or the wider 'manosphere' and right-wing voices for preying on men's insecurities and making the situation worse, but once we've blamed them, then what?

But what if we were to have a compassionate, honest and intelligent conversation about men – and one which gets to the heart of why so many of us are struggling? Because once we understand the why, then, as informed people, we can work to solve the issues (and avoid the knee-jerk, simplistic responses often spouted by the far right and far left).

This is my reason for writing this book. I'm not a fan of doing nothing. Nor am I interested in blaming certain people or segments of society for the predicament many men now face. What I am interested in is sensible conversation about what it is like to be a man, why men are struggling – and then to action! It's why my long-term commitment is to donate all profits from this book to charities and organisations supporting the wellbeing of men and boys. The good news for you, therefore, is that before you've even read this book, you've already contributed to creating better outcomes for men and boys, simply by purchasing it.

Who this book is for – and why it's for men, but not just men

This book is written first for men, and particularly for men in the UK. Perhaps, like me, you're worried for your children and want to increase your understanding of the current issues.

Perhaps you've faced your own struggles and want to

know more about why. On one level, you know your struggles are not your fault, but you're unsure about the root causes and, on a bad day, you feel inadequate and overwhelmed.

Perhaps, like the stacks of men I speak to through my podcasting and speaking work, you're confused about how you should be and what's acceptable to say. As blokes – especially blokes of a certain age in the UK – we grew up in a society where being strong and successful was a mark of our manliness. There was no space for weakness, and this can mean that instinctively, we have less time or sympathy for other men (or ourselves) when times are tough. We're also aware that, for centuries, women have faced incredible disadvantage. So, on the one hand, we know that good modern men don't bottle it up when things are shit, but on the other, we're reluctant to speak up, because we wonder whether our problems are severe enough to warrant attention, and will people even care? The more we start to think about it, the more we get bogged down in intrusive thoughts:

- What if how I really feel is too raw or may offend?
- What if my struggles are a reflection of my failings as a man? Given we blokes have been on top of the food chain for so long, to be struggling feels embarrassing.
- What if I get it wrong because I'm not used to articulating my feelings, and my foot-in-mouth moment triggers a storm I didn't intend?

Maybe it's easier to say nothing: after all, it's probably no big deal!

In reading this book, I hope you realise that if you're struggling, you're not alone, nor are you weak or a failure. The reasons why we struggle as men and why many of us are confused as to who we're supposed to be are complex. Not all men are struggling, of course, but many of us are – many more than you probably realise.

I hope that the first half of this book will help you see that your challenges are not the fault of any one person or group of people. There are multiple forces, movements and coincidences that shape how society evolves. I believe that our job as men (and as people) is to understand these forces as best we can, and then, balancing our own needs as individuals and our wider responsibilities as citizens, we have to make the wisest choices possible.

In the second part of the book, I'll be focusing on what those wise choices might be, so you can be encouraged with meaningful action points. I'll be delving into what psychological safety is, why it's so important for men and how to create it, and I'll put a spotlight on how men's communities are driving better outcomes for men today. The emergence of men's communities over the past 15 to 20 years in the UK is one of the stand-out developments for men's wellbeing and something we should be hugely encouraged by.

I'll also explore the topic of fatherhood, considering the specific challenges facing different groups of fathers, and how as men we can connect more effectively with the kids we care for in a fast-paced and complex world. And to conclude the book, I'll be talking about masculinity: how to think about it in a positive and aspirational way, without demeaning it or constraining it to a limited set of expectations.

We really can create better outcomes for ourselves, for our mates, brothers, uncles, sons, partners, and in doing so, we can indirectly create better outcomes for the women and children in our lives, too. There is a way forward for you and for society: not immediate quick fixes, but a way forward nonetheless. Some of the solutions in this book are bigger-picture ideas to stimulate your thinking for the longer term; others are practical tips that you could put into practice today.

I also hope that the women reading this book – you may have picked it up because you're worried about your sons, partners, dads, brothers, etc – will feel equipped with the knowledge to support your loved ones and steer them in directions that will enrich their lives, so the men you're worried about can get out of the rut they've been stuck in.

Why I speak, podcast and write about men

My name is Andrew Pain. I'm a TEDx and CPD-accredited speaker, podcaster, vlogger, award-winning campaigner and now I'm an author too. I'm also a dad to two grown-up daughters and three boys aged 7, 10 and 13 (at the time of writing this), which means I'm a warzone reporter, triage nurse, neurotic health and safety officer, failed caretaker, bribery and blackmailing guru, foul-mouthed taxi driver, personal football coach, maid, cook, tutor and overwhelmed slave.

If you had told me 20 years ago that today I would be a full-time international speaker, leading in my work on men's wellbeing, I would have thought you were bonkers. Twenty years ago, I was a recruitment consultant with my own one-man business, headhunting senior engineers for the world's largest engineering consultants. I ran the business from my garden shed in France (not that my clients ever knew) and during the summer months, while they probably imagined me somewhere in London, sweating in my suit, I generally worked in my underpants due to the heat (which as workwear is quite liberating: I recommend it) and my shed view was rolling vineyards, not the London skyline or a concrete wall in Croydon.

The money rolled in from my business, the sun shone (a lot), but what the heat and French wine could not mask was domestic abuse: years of it. I had no sense that what I was experiencing was domestic abuse because, at the time, I would have seen domestic abuse as something guys do to women, not the other way round. Like so many men stuck in that situation, I lived in painful ignorance (I appreciate the saying is 'blissful ignorance' but there's nothing blissful about domestic abuse, whether you recognise it or not). Over time, I was worn down by it all and my mental and physical health suffered.

After ten long years, the relationship eventually broke up, we all came back to the UK and at the same time, my business collapsed in the aftermath of the banking crisis. I eventually moved back into my parents' spare bedroom, absolutely broken in spirit, with no job, finances or prospects and, inevitably, what followed were years in the family courts battling over child contact. For those who have experienced domestic abuse, you'll know that if kids are involved, the abuse doesn't end when the relationship ends; it just evolves and changes direction. I'll refer to the family courts later in this book, but once my daughters were old enough to be out of family court procedures, I started to talk about my experiences of domestic abuse (including a TEDx talk), to see if it might be helpful for other guys experiencing abusive relationships.

I didn't have any expectations of how people might respond to me talking about domestic abuse, but what I couldn't have imagined was the sheer number of messages from women saying it had happened to their partner, son, brother, uncle, that he doesn't talk about it, but it left him in a bad way. I realised that male victims of domestic abuse are more of a hidden issue than I previously thought. This inspired me to kick-start a speaking business, primarily talking about domestic abuse, but then over the years, talking more widely about men's wellbeing and mental health.

I'm now happily remarried to a wonderful woman and we have three children together. My mental health is always under pressure from other trigger points such as finances, parenting, societal expectations, self-ambition, guilt, comparison-itis and doomscrolling (although I scroll much less than before). The more we can talk about this stuff together, the more we realise we're not alone, and the more we can support one another.

As my speaking career grew and I transitioned from part-time speaker with a supporting HR job to help pay the bills to being a full-time speaker, I started a podcast, *Men on Show*, with more than 50 episodes released and still going. The point of the podcast is to showcase the stories of everyday male heroes and the leading researchers and campaigners in the men's space. Among other things, we talk about men and PTSD, suicide, community, sobriety, addiction, sexual abuse, misandry, boys and education. I want to fill the media waves with positive stories of masculinity that will inspire the current and next generation of men. My guests are not A-list celebrities. They're ordinary guys like you and me, but many have taken small steps to make a big difference to society, and their journey should inspire us all. There's no reason why the same couldn't happen for you (although big ideas generally take *a lot* of time to get off the ground).

This book is written to address the physical and mental health crisis facing men. I hope it will be of value to all men, regardless of cultural outlook, sexuality or gender preference, and also to the women who have men they care about, whether the women are sisters, mothers, partners, aunts, neighbours or work colleagues.

It was once asked of me during a conference I was speaking at: 'Can women really help in solving the issues faced by men?'

To which I responded: 'One hundred per cent *yes*!'

Just as male action and allyship is key to solving the many challenges that women and girls still grapple with, the same is true for women and girls supporting the men and boys they love. If you're a woman reading this book, I'm honoured. Please do stand with us in solidarity and let's address the issues we face as people together. We're better together than apart. It's hugely powerful when one group of people speaks up for another. There are too many people trying to divide us.

The three questions this book is going to answer

This book is organised around three key questions:

1. Are there issues for men today? (And if so, says who?)
2. Why are there issues for men?
3. How do we solve the issues?

Chapter 1 investigates the evidence around the six most discussed indicators when assessing men's wellbeing: suicide, homelessness, the prison population, education, loneliness and life expectancy. It's an important place to start, because some people understandably feel a bit cynical about the reality of men's suffering. So, rather than ignore that sentiment, I think it's helpful to reflect on what these six indicators may communicate about men's struggles today. To do this, I'll be drawing on global research, the views of my podcast guests and my own lived experience.

Chapters 2 to 6 form Part 1 of the book and they explore the second key question: why are there issues for men? I examine a range of issues that have conspired to make a difficult mix for men. In these chapters, I'll focus mainly on UK experiences but also bring in studies and perspectives from around the world.

Chapter 2 looks at the impact of sweeping economic changes during the last century (from automation to austerity) and how these have affected men's experiences today, particularly working-class men.

In Chapter 3, I'll examine the pace of cultural change (such as modern dating, the #MeToo movement, falling birth rates) and whether or not gendered stereotypes have kept up with these changes.

Chapter 4 turns to the sensitive topic of how men are talked about within society, from negative media messaging and toxic masculinity to political laziness. Why are these things a problem? And without scoring points for certain political parties (while having a dig at others), I'll consider whether men's challenges have been largely ignored by successive governments.

In Chapter 5, I switch attention to technology and the impact of the digital world on men: from online pornography to the manosphere, gambling and social media. Can we really pass some of the blame for men's suffering onto the digital world?

Chapter 6 concludes the first part of the book by focusing on male health. You may have heard rumblings about declining testosterone levels (most people haven't), but how serious is the decline? Is that good news or bad news? And if it's bad news, how do we stop the decline?

In each of these chapters, as well as unpacking the issues, I've also included my thoughts on how to address them, so even before we get to answering the third key question in Part 2 ('How do we solve the issues?') you'll already have plenty of ideas from Part 1!

The second part of the book showcases solutions to help men move forward. You'll find separate chapters on psychological safety, men's communities, fatherhood and redefining masculinity.

If there is one concept that could positively transform our workplaces and communities, it's psychological safety. In Chapter 7, I explain why it's important for everyone, regardless of gender, but how it's particularly relevant for those men who may have been brought up to believe that a real man gets on with it, takes no shit and doesn't make a fuss. Shifting from old restrictive stereotypes to psychological safety is a big step, so if we're going to make the effort to take it, we should first understand why it's so important and then how to create it.

In Chapter 8, I focus on men's communities. These communities have exploded across the UK, with men finding friendship, adventure and safe spaces where they can talk more openly. Men's communities save lives and drive better mental and physical health outcomes for men, so if you're feeling isolated, I hope you'll feel inspired by the selection of communities I describe in this chapter and that you connect with a men's community near you. And if you are thinking of starting your own initiative, then the stories of the male community builders I share should give you some useful starting points so you can get going. Expect to be inspired by men who thought 'Why not?'... and had a go at it.

Chapter 9 puts the spotlight on fatherhood. If the next generation of men need role models, then the current generation of men need to deliver the goods as informed and compassionate leaders. This chapter will help you to better understand the challenges faced by different groups of dads, so we can all help them to be the best role models for their families. I'll also reflect on how to be the best role models to the children in our care, whether we're biological dads, stepfathers, uncles or concerned neighbours.

In my final chapter, I look at redefining masculinity. If traditional stereotypes of what a man is and does are no longer fit for purpose, then what next? In this chapter, I will pick apart masculinity to help you think about how we can create a narrative which is positive and real, and which allows men to think for themselves about what kind of people they choose to be.

Finding inspiration and reaching out

I'm writing this book because, aside from my dad worries, I'm inspired by:

- three joyful, mischievous, energetic sons and two larger-than-life, dynamic and comical daughters
- the dads I know in my community, working tirelessly to be a provider, protector, lover and father to the families they serve

- the amazing campaigners, unsung heroes and researchers I meet through my speaking work and podcast
- the wonderful female allies who stand shoulder to shoulder with men. (Please keep up your good work and don't lose heart. You're very much needed in today's divided society. As men we need you, even if we don't say it enough)
- my wonderful wife, talented sisters, steadfastly loyal mum and aunts, and three sisters-in-law.

As worried as I am, these people fuel my motivation as a speaker, writer and podcaster. I want this book to be a unifier, creating balanced debate on potentially contentious topics, bringing men, women, people together in addressing the issues men face in society, because men's issues are everyone's issues.

And finally, before we get started, if you're reading this book because you're struggling and you want to feel hopeful, please do reach out for help. Don't suffer alone because you're not alone (even if it feels like you are). Modern society is fast paced so it's easy to get caught up with our own stuff and we miss other people who might be struggling, even people we know well – but rest assured, as people, we do genuinely care.

Most of us want to help. It's an honour to help. We just need to know you're struggling because we won't necessarily guess that you are.

And if you do happen to reach out to someone who seems a bit flaky, please don't take it personally or lose faith in humanity. They might be struggling themselves. Instead, reach out again to someone else. There are plenty of good people in society who are ready to help today.

However bad life feels today, and however messy your mess is, there is always a way forward. Don't give up.

1 Are there issues for men today? (And if so, says who?)

Go check out the news in the mainstream media, scroll your social media feeds and, just to be sure, ask ChatGPT the following questions:

1. Do women and girls still face inequality and disadvantage in the 21st century?
2. Is the world today a safer place for women and girls?
3. Is misogyny on the decline?

Then grab a seat and coffee, take a deep breath and prepare for the avalanche of data that comes back at you: the horrific lived-experience stories from women and girls that will make your blood boil, and the pleas for resources to tackle violence against women and girls. It seems obvious to me that while some progress has been made in achieving equality for women and girls, we've still got a long way to go. Looking at the world with my Western, liberal, heterosexual man-lens, it sometimes feels as if we're still in the dark ages. It's partly why the conversation around the struggles of men and women can be so divisive.

So, let's be clear on two things. First, this book is about men. Second, the work in creating equality for women and girls is nowhere near complete and it's why I'm occasionally asked: 'How bad can it be for men, when things are still so bad for women?' I think this is a fair question, so in this chapter I'm going to investigate six serious issues: suicide, homelessness, prison, education, loneliness and life expectancy. I've chosen these topics because, when men's challenges are discussed within media and political circles, it's generally these six that are drawn upon to justify the concern. Taken together, I think it's crystal clear that large groups of men are really struggling, so if you're one of them, you're certainly not alone.

The tragedy of suicide

Suicide is a global tragedy and sobering reminder that for all the progress we've made within modern society, not everyone is benefiting. Wherever we look in the world, far more men die by suicide than women. In the US, for example, in research highlighted by the American Institute for Boys and Men (Reeves & Secker 2024), men are four times more likely to die from suicide than women, with figures currently reaching close to 50,000 deaths per year (which is more than deaths from road traffic accidents).

In the UK, men are three times more likely than women to fall victim to suicide, particularly men in the 45- to 49-year-old age bracket, men who are disadvantaged and men who've just experienced a relationship breakdown (Samaritans 2025, Centre for Social Justice 2025, Wilson et al 2025). It's a national scandal that if you live in the most deprived areas of England, you're twice as likely to die from suicide than if you live in the most affluent areas (Kirk-Wade 2025) and for all the campaigns in the past 10–15 years, urging us men to seek help, to talk about our troubles and not bottle them up, the numbers of us still dying from suicide are not yet decreasing.

Men use more lethal means to complete suicide than

women, such as guns and hanging (Berardelli & Rogante 2022) and there is an argument voiced by some that women *attempt* suicide in similar numbers to men, therefore suicide is as much as a problem for women as it is for men: the difference is in the number of *deaths* by suicide. While we should never lose sight of the number of women who attempt and die by suicide, the reality is that we lose far more men to suicide than women, which to me suggests that there are serious problems in society for men. Steve Phillip is a leading UK campaigner whose mission is to create a zero-suicide society following the tragic death of his son Jordan. He was the second guest to appear on my podcast, and during our conversation, he was clear that most suicide deaths are preventable with the right societal, workplace and community infrastructure in place.

So, while we can understandably feel defeated and hopeless in the face of the never-ending stream of tragedy, we should also be mindful that what Steve Phillip is fighting for (a zero-suicide society) is not an idealistic utopia. In Finland, for example, they've halved the number of people dying by suicide each year through the establishment of a National Suicide Prevention Programme and ongoing action over many years (Bryant 2024).

In the UK, it is encouraging to see suicide highlighted as a particular focus within the recent UK Men's Health Strategy, announced in November 2025. Action points within the strategy include: fostering partnerships with sports and popular culture platforms, improving men's access to health services and the support of community-based suicide prevention programmes. All well and good so far, but there is a problem when we think about the scale of the issue. A promised investment of £3.6 million over a three-year period really is a drop in the ocean.

Homelessness: it's complex, but men fare worse

You may have heard that 85 per cent of homeless people across the world are men, but the homelessness data is complex. I was employed for ten years by a charity whose work is focused on reducing homelessness, so I do know a thing or two about it and, in the UK at least, there are three different types of homelessness:

1. **Rough sleeping:** In the streets, doorways of shops, cardboard shelters under bridges, park benches, in a tent in a field, in your car or a public building that is not built for habitation (such as car parks and stairwells). You have no fixed shelter or a suitable building to live in: you're surviving with whatever you can find.
2. **Temporary accommodation:** Hostels, bed and breakfast accommodation or local hotels, generally paid for by local government and the third sector. You have a roof over your head, at least, but it's definitely *not* the Ritz. Forget room service, forget a spa or leisure facilities and forget a wide-ranging breakfast buffet. Temporary accommodation is extremely basic and can drag on for months.
3. **Sofa surfing:** Staying indefinitely with your friends/family, moving from address to address. You might be camping out in a spare room on a mattress/airbed for a while, or on a sofa sharing the space with your hosts. You're in a house at least but it's short term, week by week and you're likely to be moving between multiple addresses to spread the load on your network.

In the UK, 85 per cent of rough sleepers are men, but it's believed that there are more female sofa surfers in the UK than male, while 60 per cent of people in temporary accommodation in the UK are women (Statista Research Department

2025, Shelter 2021). But across the world, 70 per cent of homeless people appear to be men, with numbers varying from country to country, as well as the national definitions of what homelessness is (OECD 2023). That so many more men are homeless and rough sleepers than women when, economically speaking, we've been at the top of the food chain for so long, is a paradox I'll come back to in Chapter 2.

Imprisonment: an overwhelmingly male issue

If 95 per cent of people in prison globally are men, doesn't this prove that we're more violent and prone to criminal behaviour than women? Maybe as a man, with my XY chromosomes, I've still got it in me to be a badass gangster or maybe there's a better question we could ask:

- What's the journey a man takes to arrive at a point of criminal behaviour?

In England, if you live in one of the ten most deprived areas of the country, your risk of experiencing a custodial sentence is ten times higher than if you grow up in one of the ten most affluent areas (Cardiff University 2022). Of course, we all have a choice on whether or not to live a life of crime, but your experience of poverty and deprivation has a tenfold impact on your level of risk as a future criminal. In Scotland, there is a similar pattern, with nearly half the prison population coming from the nation's most deprived postcodes (Families Outside 2023). Poverty, men and prison: they go hand in hand, because if you examine household poverty within a deprived postcode, what you face can include:

- a lack of local employment opportunities and economic barriers that prevent you travelling further to access better jobs (due to fuel poverty and commuting expenses)

- a long-term lack of purpose or hope within the household or family, due to a lack of employment
- financial despair, day-to-day debt and, in some cases, ongoing risk of eviction, all of which combine to create instability
- a chaotic or dysfunctional home where, for young people growing up, there is increased risk of one of the caregivers having a substance abuse issue
- no or minimal qualifications
- a lack of local facilities and things to do, such as youth groups/centres, so boredom is rife and your opportunities to develop your skills are reduced. This is accompanied by a lack of safe, green space because across Europe, the more deprived the postcode, the less access to green space you'll have (European Environment Agency 2022).

I've barely scratched the surface of a mountain of disadvantages you'll face if you grow up within a deprived postcode – and yet for men at least, we'll still be carrying the societal expectation of being a provider.

Men convicted of crime have made choices that have led them to where they are, but if 95 per cent of people in prison are men, and if living in a deprived postcode has such a marked effect on your chances of experiencing a custodial sentence, it's clear that there are external factors that put many men at increased risk of falling into crime and being jailed: factors that are not their fault or of their choosing.

It doesn't take a genius to work out that once men have been convicted and served their sentence, what waits for them on the other side is more poverty, homelessness, unemployment and social isolation, all of which lead them back into crime. It's a vicious cycle and when over half of prisoners in the UK have literacy skills below the expected levels of an average 11-year-old, it's not surprising that with the added stigma of having a criminal record, 70 per cent of people remain unemployed six months after release from prison (Ofsted & His Majesty's Inspectorate of Prisons 2022, Ministry of Justice 2025).

- 95 per cent tells a story of male despair and dysfunction.
- 95 per cent is driven largely by external circumstances rather than rotten male genes.
- 95 per cent is an indicator that not all men benefit from their so-called privilege of being born a man.

Education: it's about boys *and* men

Things have quickly changed in the world of university education. In the UK, in the 1990s, less than half of university graduates were female (Advance HE 2025), but now 54 per cent of graduates are female and the gap is increasing. There have been similar changes in the US too, as evidenced by the Pew Research Center (Hurst 2024). On the one hand, it may feel like random data and maybe we should just celebrate the fact that after years of struggle, we're seeing women graduate in greater numbers than men. However, as more women than men graduate, according to the influential 'Lost Boys' report, the gender pay gap in the UK has reversed for the 16- to 24-year-old age group (Centre for Social Justice 2025), and far more men in their twenties and early thirties are still living at home with their parents in comparison with women (Clark 2025). This indicates that falling education attainment levels for males are not something to shrug off as 'no big deal' and may be part of the reason why so many of us men seem unable to live independently in our twenties and early thirties. It's a cause for concern, for reasons I'll explore in Chapter 2.

It may be that the educational rot has set in long before the age of 18. Research from Cambridge University Press &

Assessment found that in the UK, females outperform males in every regular school subject – barring maths – at every school age (Moran 2024) and in terms of classroom behaviour, boys are twice as likely to be excluded from school than girls (Department for Education 2025). The reality of exclusion includes social stigma, shame, falling even further behind in your education, loss of friendship networks and loneliness, all of which lead to destructive behaviour. This in turn increases the chances of isolation, poor mental health and, in the long term, prison. And just in case you were wondering, it's the least privileged boys who fare the worst, with disadvantaged boys being five times more likely to be excluded from school than advantaged boys (Centre for Social Justice 2025).

From suicide to prison and education, it's clear that social inequality and poverty are at the root of many of the issues that men wrestle with today. Even for boys who are not excluded nor disadvantaged, behaviour is more of a challenge within a traditional classroom environment. In a survey of American teachers, while 50 per cent observed that boys struggled to sit still and pay attention in class, only 18 per cent observed the same issue with girls (Heubeck 2025).

Boredom at school... I remember it so clearly and see it today in my sons' experiences: learning about stuff I didn't care about, spending hour after hour inside, not knowing what the teacher was going on about because I couldn't pay attention. What I needed was more physical activity and time outside, but in the UK, even with what we now know about the differing needs of girls and boys, and about the impact of the testosterone boost due to male puberty, more than two million children are doing less than 30 minutes of physical activity each day. The government recommends just two hours of physical education to be taught each week at secondary schools, but not only is this nowhere near enough, it's not enforceable and, added to this, the number of PE hours being taught are actually decreasing due to staffing issues (Roan

2025). No wonder so many young males struggle to sit still in class. Poor fellas! I really do feel their pain.

The question of how to create an educational system that best supports the needs of boys and girls is a complex one, but one thing is certain: right now, large groups of boys are struggling within the education system as it is, not just in the US or the UK but across Europe, and this struggle appears to be affecting their opportunities as they become adults. In a fast-paced and uncertain world, where the number of jobs in traditionally male industries such as agriculture and manufacturing has dramatically dropped, if young men have hopes of being independent and supporting a family, then they have to make the best of their educational opportunities. But the data suggests this isn't happening. Unless we address this issue, we can expect to see increasing numbers of disillusioned, bored young males, impoverished, with low aspiration and little trust in society: in fact, when you look at modern society, it's already in motion.

The rise of *kudokushi* and male loneliness

Kudokushi: you've probably guessed it's a Japanese term, but I'm assuming it's not one you've heard of.

Most people haven't but remember this term – you'll be seeing more of it in years to come. It's being talked about in Japan, South Korea, Italy and the UK. It's a growing phenomenon and refers to a 'loneliness death', where the body of the deceased person is not found until months after they died.

Kudokushi deaths are on the rise, with close to 70,000 annual deaths in Japan alone and 10,000 in the UK. And when it comes to the gender split, you're twice as likely to die a *kudokushi* death in Japan as a man than you are a woman (Huaxia 2024) and nearly three times as likely to die a *kudokushi* death in the UK as a man than a woman (Coffey 2024). We're in the early days of capturing data on *kudokushi*, but while it affects both men and women, the picture so far suggests it's a bigger issue for men.

In the UK and beyond, loneliness is a growing problem due to a toxic combination of social factors:

- the legacy of austerity across Europe since 2010, with literally billions of pounds of funding cut for social and community programmes
- the impact of Covid-19, which increased social isolation across the globe
- the rise of home and remote working
- bad technology habits, with people of all ages glued to their phones and screens
- a fast-paced, 24/7 society, which means people have become more impatient than 40 or 50 years ago, so we have less time for building and maintaining friendships than we once did
- falling marriage and birth rates.

There's nothing surprising in this list nor is it surprising that loneliness appears to be getting worse for men. In the US, the percentage of men who said they had no close friends in the early 1990s was 3 per cent and now it's 15 per cent (Cox 2021) – a fivefold increase in a relatively short space of time. This corresponds with data showing that the number of hours American young men (aged 18 to 29) spend alone each day has increased from 4.1 hours in 2003 to 6.6 hours in 2023, according to the American Time Use Survey (Rampell 2025).

'Man-keeping' is another new term in the modern vocabulary, referring to the fact that men are increasingly reliant on their female partner for emotional support, while the same does not appear to be true in reverse. This corresponds with research showing that post divorce, men are more likely to experience loneliness than women because they're less likely to have a social circle of their own to draw on (Wright et al 2019). Men's mental health charity and thinktank Movember refers to a 'male friendship recession', with nearly half of men they surveyed reporting they couldn't talk about a problem to a friend (Block 2024).

Loneliness ruins your physical and mental health, whoever you are. I've been there and experienced it years ago during my first term at university (which I still regard as some of the worst months of my life). It destroys your confidence and becomes a vicious cycle because you feel less equipped to take the steps you need to in order to stop being lonely – such as trying new things, meeting new people and making yourself vulnerable.

The life expectancy gap

There is no question that women live longer than men. They have done for centuries. Even before the 1930s when, historically, so many women were lost to childbirth (thus reducing women's life expectancy overall), women still lived longer than men. But should we simply accept the life expectancy gap? And what if it's getting worse?

In the UK, the life expectancy gap between men and women is four years (ONS 2025a). In the US, the life expectancy gender gap grew from a 4.8-year difference in 2010 to 5.8 years in 2021 (Yan et al 2023). Globally, you can see similar life expectancy gaps of around five years within the African continent, growing to a nearly ten-year gap in parts of Eastern Europe (Dattani 2025). The reasons are varied, but key factors include:

- **Covid-19:** Based on data from 73 countries, an estimated 300,000 more men died from Covid-19 than women, according to a review of data in the *Bulletin of the World Health Organization* (Ramírez-Soto et al 2021). This spiked the numbers of male deaths when looking at data from the early 2020s.

- **Deaths of despair:** Including suicide, drug overdose and alcohol abuse, deaths of despair affect men in greater numbers than women. In 2019 for example, globally, an estimated two million men died from alcohol abuse in comparison with 600,000 women (World Health Organization 2024).
- **Riskier employment:** Agriculture, forestry, fishing, mining, quarrying, construction, roofing, iron and steel works: these professions are 'dirty and dangerous' jobs (DAD jobs), carrying a higher risk of serious injury or death and dominated by men. Given the nature of the work, it's not surprising that in the UK, for example, 95 per cent of people who died in 2023 to 2024 due to workplace accidents were men (Health and Safety Executive 2025).
- **Health outcomes:** Men generally experience worse health outcomes for diseases such as cardiovascular disease, lung cancer, liver disease and diabetes than women (Fenney & Raleigh 2024).

Why these issues mustn't be ignored

Suicide, homelessness, prison, education, loneliness, life expectancy: six key indicators suggesting that not all is well for men, and that in spite of a historic privilege within the group of people that is 'men', there is enormous disadvantage too.

- If we ignore these issues, then we accept preventable human suffering.
- If we ignore these issues, then others with darker intentions won't and they'll play on the undercurrent of resentment and pain.
- If we ignore these issues, then we accept the ripple effect

across families and communities caused by suicide, abuse, violence, homelessness and poverty.

I'm not prepared to accept these things. I doubt you are either.

So, if we can agree that men are genuinely facing issues that warrant attention and resources, that advocating for women's equality and men's wellbeing can be done at the same time, and if we can agree that a step forward for one group is not a step backward for the other, then two key questions must be explored so we pursue the right courses of action as individuals, communities and as a society.

1. Why are there issues for men?
2. How do we solve the issues?

These two questions form Parts 1 and 2 of this book. In the next chapter, I'll dive into the reasons why there are issues for men, starting with the seismic changes in society during the past 70–80 years.

Part 1

Why are there issues for men?

2 Not all men are privileged

> "Imagine a woman who goes to private school, whose dad is a stockbroker and mother a barrister. She goes to Oxbridge and straight into a job in the city. Is she less privileged than a black or white working-class lad from a council estate in south London?"

Mark Brooks, OBE, director of policy and communications at the independent think-tank Centre for Policy Research on Men and Boys, national ambassador for International Men's Day (UK) and founding trustee of the Association of Male Health and Wellbeing (previously the Men and Boys Coalition) from the Men on Show *podcast, episode 5*

I was bursting with pride, heart racing, key in hand: this was *the* moment I became a man. I was 23 years old.

For anyone else, it was a mediocre, two-bedroom, ex-council flat on a bland side road, situated between Balham and Tooting Bec in south London. It's not even as if I owned it or had sole occupancy – I was renting it with my mate. But having moved to the capital for my first job after graduating, I now had my own place, for which I was (jointly) responsible. This was the stand-out moment in my life, when I felt I'd transitioned from boy to man. I truly registered it at the time, and nearly 30 years later, I still remember the moment I first unlocked that front door and entered *my* flat.

Growing up, I'd never doubted that I'd be able to rent a flat by my early twenties. As a milestone, it gave me a new sense of maturity, to the point where I felt different: older, wiser, standing on my own two feet for the first time, no longer reliant on my parents (or the state) and working a job that paid the rent and my bills. Expectations can make or break us. On the one hand, they can help us to dig deeper when we need to, but on the other, they can create extreme dissatisfaction when they're not met. My expectations that I'd find somewhere I could afford to rent and then purchase a property in my twenties felt ordinary and achievable – and both expectations were met within the timescale I envisaged. I didn't expect a life of dripping wealth, but the milestones of university, independence, home ownership, marriage, fatherhood, stable finances felt reasonable to expect as a white, middle-class chap growing up in the 1980s and 1990s.

But oh, how the world has changed for our young men today!

My 'reasonable' milestones must now seem like pie-in-the-sky for most of Generation Z and if you want to understand why so many men are struggling, it's important to first consider how the world has changed for men, turning once achievable milestones into pure fantasy.

In this chapter, I'm going to examine the economic changes that have transformed former industrial areas in the UK, squashing communities and eliminating any realistic hope for working-class men to live up to the 'provider' male stereotype. In the next chapter, I'll consider the additional impact for men of cultural changes, such as the #MeToo movement, falling birth rates and a changing dating scene. You may have felt angered by men 'behaving badly', or the 'deadbeat dads' you hear about and the wave of 'toxic masculinity' on display in society, but the reasons why men are struggling are complex, and understanding the breadth of those reasons is key to forming an intelligent and compassionate response to the challenges we face.

Men and the industrial decline

Head back in a time machine to 1970s Britain and the male-dominated industries of manufacturing, agriculture and construction contributed more than 40 per cent of the UK's economic output. Life was tough for the men who laboured day to day in the grime and smoke. You didn't get rich doing manual work – it was dirty, dangerous and offered minimal opportunities for career advancement, but you had a stable job for life, or at least while you could physically work. Jump back into that same time machine and return to today and you'll find the contribution of these male-dominated industries towards UK economic output has shrunk to just 16 per cent – and with that decline has come the loss of literally millions of jobs: millions of male jobs (Centre for Social Justice 2025).

To put this into perspective, in 1970 there were 7.7 million jobs in UK manufacturing, accounting for 29 per cent of UK employment, but by 2021, that number had fallen to 2.5 million jobs and 8 per cent respectively (Cominetti et al 2022). It's easy to skip over the data when our world is awash with so much of it, so let's be clear: these statistics tell a profoundly negative story for working-class men, in terms both of economics and of social cohesion.

The most obvious impact is a massive drop in the availability of employment opportunities for men and particularly those with low levels of formal education. Before the decline in agricultural and manufacturing employment, if you left school with no qualifications, you could still find stable work and with it a sense of purpose, pride and an ability, of sorts, to feed, clothe and house a family. While it would be naive of me to romanticise what was no doubt an extremely tough life as a manual labourer in 1950s Britain, it's fair to say that a working-class man with limited qualifications at least had a role in society and an income that meant he could provide something.

But with the rise of automation in the 20th century, and a move away from manufacturing into a service-based economy, there has been a staggering loss of employment for working-class men, and what has followed has been searing poverty in former industrial areas, resulting in large groups of men who are lost, disconnected from society and struggling to understand their purpose as men any more. As I discussed in Chapter 1, poverty hugely increases your risk of experiencing a custodial sentence (which further reduces your employability) and your risk of dying by suicide, while also decreasing your life expectancy by a jaw-dropping ten years (ONS 2022).

Aside from the obvious economic impact of deindustrialisation, there is a social consequence, too. From the mining pits to the steel works and car factories, at the very centre of these industries were thriving communities of men, from sporting clubs to music clubs and men's working and social clubs. These communities provided a life-saving break from the bleakness of factory life, where men bonded, excelled, competed, worked and played together.

The Grimethorpe Colliery Band, one of the finest British brass bands, was founded in 1917 by miners in the Yorkshire pits, one of many such brass bands with a proud, working-class tradition. The Treorchy Male Choir, formed in the Welsh mining valleys, was one of many Welsh male choirs to emerge from the soot and muck of pit life. The undeniably best and most prestigious football team in world history, Arsenal Football Club (I'm a bit biased), was formed by workers from a Royal Arsenal munitions factory in Woolwich in 1886, while West Ham United was set up by workers from Thames Steel. These are just a handful of many such examples, and as communities of men, they embodied the discipline, collaboration and competitive spirit honed within the pits, factories and steel works. They gave men a sense of belonging, identity and creative joy, uniting entire communities around shared goals and rivalries.

But as the factories shut and the pits closed, not only did this wreak economic havoc on the families who lived and worked in these areas, it also wreaked havoc on the fabric of community life. In a time of desperation, fear and hopelessness, many of the support networks that had previously held men together rusted away, along with the bleak ghost towns and industrial remnants of abandoned factories. We can't turn back time, of course, and glamourising British industrial life is misleading and unproductive. But we can move forward, accepting that despite the historic privilege of being born male, large groups of British men, particularly working-class British men, are really struggling, that it's not just in the UK this has happened and expecting men to simply man up or get better at talking about their feelings isn't going to cut it.

In America, in the 1950s, only 2 per cent of men of prime working age (between the ages of 24 and 54) were not employed or looking for work (Dokoupil & Finn 2023). Today, that percentage of disconnected men has quadrupled to 10 per cent (Lee 2025). Added to this, since the 1950s, the population size of America has also doubled, which means in terms of sheer numbers, there has been a staggering increase of prime working-age men, both out of work and not looking for work.

It's no surprise that in the Equimundo 'State of American Men 2025' report, 75 per cent of men surveyed said they feel it's much harder for their generation to be financially secure than their father's generation. They no longer feel able to bring home the bacon and put food on the table as they saw their fathers do, and with financial instability and a lack of hope come despair and apathy. The same survey found that financial instability increased the likelihood of men experiencing suicidal thoughts by more than 16 times. As the UK, US and other nations have globalised and deindustrialised in the 20th and early 21st centuries, there have been economic winners and economic losers, and many working-class men have lost.

Lightbulb moment: Men who are disadvantaged

> While, traditionally, men have had a historic privilege from being born male, within the group that is men there are huge numbers who are greatly disadvantaged and any talk of 'privilege' is frankly insulting.

To make matters worse, another issue has emerged in most developed countries. It's a complex problem that is difficult to solve. It's been festering for decades and seems to be a particular problem for men. You may have heard of it... the housing crisis!

Men and the housing crisis

Wherever you go in Europe, it's the same: soaring property prices, rents going up and a severe shortage of affordable homes. In the UK, in the early 1970s, house prices were typically 3.5 times your annual salary, whereas today they're often eight to nine times your annual earnings. Across Europe, while average disposable incomes have increased by just 17 per cent between 2005 and 2023, rents have gone up by 34 per cent and house prices by 76 per cent (Koessl 2025).

You may wonder why housing has become such a massive issue. The roots of the problem are widespread, including seeing housing as a commodity or asset rather than a place to live, a lack of investment in new, affordable and social housing, and the privatisation of existing public or non-profit housing, which has shrunk the housing stock of affordable homes across many European countries.

I bought my first house in Carshalton, Surrey at the age of 27 and borrowed just over four times my annual salary to do it, with no deposit required, securing a 105 per cent loan (the extra bit on top of the full house price loan was to clear a few debts). For me, purchasing a property and fulfilling my inner need to provide was far easier than it is for men today.

In a report last year, the Institute for Fiscal Studies found that while 55 per cent of 24- to 35-year-olds in the UK were homeowners in 1997, by 2017 that percentage had dropped to 35 per cent (Brader 2024). Even if you have a well-paying job, it's almost impossible to achieve a house purchase without the bank of Mum and Dad, and if you're a working-class man who is either not employed or employed in unstable or low-paid roles, and you're not likely to have cash-rich parents, then home ownership is fantasyland. You could suggest that a man in this situation rents instead because, once upon a time, most people rented quite happily, so get over it. But just as house prices across the UK and Europe have shot up, so have rental prices.

While the housing crisis obviously affects both men and women, in a 2025 Statista report on the gender breakdown of adults still living with their parents in 2023, it was found that 47 per cent of males over the age of 24 still live with their parents (in comparison with just 29 per cent of women). For those over the age of 30, 16 per cent of men still live with their parents in comparison with just 5 per cent of women (Clark 2025).

The truth is that it's difficult today to set up a home and provide, and yet the stereotype of a man as provider still holds firm.

This stereotype is as old as the hills but as clear as day. Its basic premise is this:

Your job as a man is to provide for your partner/wife and family, and the more you can provide, the more of a man you are, and the more likely it is that you'll find a suitable partner. The less you can provide, the less of a man you are, and if you have a female partner who can provide more than you can, then you're not much of a man, so pull yourself together and make something of yourself.

Men and austerity

There's an inevitable equation that the UK experienced in full. It goes like this:

Global banking crisis + Massive banking bailout = Austerity = Suffering for those at the lowest end of society

If you're struggling today, none of the above factors are your fault, but they're part of why so many of us struggle. Austerity meant cutback after cutback, where social groups and projects that held communities together like glue were evaporated, and none more so than youth projects. We hear a lot today about the need for positive male role models, or of purposeless, toxic young males in need of guidance, or of absent fathers, shirking their responsibilities. I hear people asking questions in my workshops/talks, such as:

- Where are all the good men?
- Why aren't there more male guardian angels in society?

The truth is that there have always been plenty of male angels in our communities, but prior to austerity, those angels had a bit of help, not just from God, but from local government too. More than a thousand local government-funded youth centres across the UK have shut because of austerity, resulting in the loss of thousands of talented youth workers and hundreds of places to be, with positive things to do, staffed by positive role models.

Research by the public service union UNISON found that four out of every ten councils in the UK no longer operate any youth centres, something that is linked to increased knife crime in those areas, increased school exclusions, worsening mental health and young people at greater risk of gang involvement because they're bored and hanging around the streets. For disadvantaged communities where there is a lack of green space and widespread poverty, this is particularly devastating for young people, and it adds to the narrative that no one cares, so look out for yourself first and foremost (UNISON 2024).

Austerity was not your fault, nor was the banking crisis, nor the housing crisis, nor deindustrialisation. But these things may well have had a negative social and economic impact on your experience as a man, while the notion of your provider role and of your worth being measured by material success have never been so absurd, but still hold firm.

We also need action from government to robustly tackle the housing crisis, understanding that the root causes of the crisis are complex, they've been long in the making, they long preceded the rise in the number of migrants crossing the channel on boats (so don't blame UK housing issues on immigrants) and it will require more than just promises to increase the supply of affordable homes.

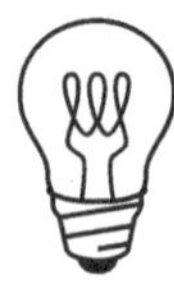

Lightbulb moment: Why government investment and action are needed

We need to see action from government – action that is specifically man-focused – to restore our belief and hope that wider society cares about struggling men. We should not fear or apologise for putting aside budget for specifically male causes because every pound we invest in men is a pound for improving society as a whole. I'm heartened by the discussion around a British industrial strategy to revitalise former industrial heartlands, for example. It's been a long time in the making and still has a long way to go, including how to ensure that the job creation is targeted towards those who have been left behind, but the discussion of the strategy is encouraging nonetheless and a step in the right direction.

3 The world has changed – but stereotypes haven't

> "Thirty years ago, we had stronger family units, we had bigger families, we had communities, so we were more supported. We had more people that knew us. We had a family doctor that knew us well. There's less support now. We're more isolated. We're more disconnected than we've ever been, weirdly, because digitally we're more connected than ever."

Daniel Glyde, transformational coach working exclusively with men, from the Men on Show *podcast, episode 40*

Do you ever have those moments when a certain sound or sight catapults you back in time to when your life felt simpler, easier, happier?

For me, it's clips from 1980s TV or the theme tunes for programmes like *Blind Date*, *The A Team*, *Bergerac*, *Dynasty* and *Dallas*. We'd gather around our TV as a family (it was the only 'screen' in the household) and these programmes would generate so much conversation and wonder in our house. These were precious moments, and today the memories make the hairs on my neck stand up. Where did all the time go? It only feels like yesterday. Life was just so much better before... but before when? And was life genuinely better in the 1980s than it is now?

It's easy to forget that these were also the years of the miners' strike, social upheaval and individuals such as Jimmy Savile and Mohamed Al Fayed running riot, abusing people on a mass scale while too many people knew, looked on and thought better of tackling it due to self-preservation. Life was not the dreamy utopia we sometimes remember it to be, and not all progress is bad, but society has evolved rapidly. As well as the economic impact of deindustrialisation and austerity discussed in Chapter 2, other sweeping changes have had a profound impact on the experiences of men.

In this chapter, I'll explore how dating has evolved, the consequences of the #MeToo movement and the reality of falling birth rates, while also unpacking the traditional man code stereotypes and why they're no longer fit for purpose. If there's one thing to take away from this chapter, it's to consider what your own man code looks like and whether it truly serves you well, given how times have changed.

Dating and the loss of community spaces

Dating in the 1980s and 1990s was a bit different in comparison with today. No Tinder, no internet or dating sites, no online pornography, no phones with cameras to record the mishaps, no sextortion, no fear of accusations if you screwed up: it was more straightforward back in my day.

As my testosterone levels soared in my teens and my world became fixated on girls, I knew that if I wanted a girlfriend, I'd need to put myself in situations where I would naturally meet girls. I'd also need to make something of myself, to compete and excel at stuff. I'd need something to offer, in terms of personality, resources and skills. There'd be no quick fixes, and I'd need to learn the art of charm, respect and being an all-round gentleman. Anything less would simply prolong being single. It was all quite healthy stuff for a developing, heterosexual teenager. Dating wasn't easy, but dating shouldn't be too easy!

Looking back, mistakes were made, but without the mass humiliation of social media exposure or pictures taken in awkward situations, without the danger of false accusations that could ruin my life. And without the danger that just maybe, the girl I was falling for was not actually the beautiful and sincere stunner I thought she was, but 'she' was actually 'he' and an online scammer based overseas with one simple intention: to lure me into their web of lies, so they could blackmail me for cash. These weren't issues in my dating days, and in the periods when I was single, I had plenty of other social stuff going on, so there was always hope, because I was always meeting people (girls) in natural settings, from church youth to orchestras, to the musical performances each year at the mixed comprehensive school I attended.

Dating was more straightforward, even for a total novice who looked much younger than his actual age. Sure, there were a few stormy days here and there, but for young men today, from teens and to adults, dating is less of a rainy walk in the park: it's a minefield in a shitstorm. No wonder so many men give up and watch porn instead or seek comfort in an AI partner.

There are a few aspects to why dating has changed and how this has made the whole experience quite miserable and unsatisfying. One of the changes is due to a word we've already explored in Chapter 2: austerity! As a legacy of austerity, a failing economy and the impact of Covid isolation, it's not just youth services that have taken a battering: at the same time, we've also seen the loss of pubs, theatres, community spaces, discos and nightclubs. According to the British Beer and Pub Association, the UK has lost nearly 16,000 pubs in the 21st century (Thatcher 2025), the rate of losses speeding up from austerity onwards. At the same time, since austerity measures kicked into gear, the UK has also lost half its nightclubs (Business Rescue Expert 2025). Those pub and nightclub losses represent a staggering reduction in places where people naturally mixed, matched and moved on.

Between 2017 and 2022, nearly 50 community spaces (not including youth centres) were lost in London alone, with similar community space losses across the UK, according to the Foundation for Future London (Glass 2024). And of course, with UK councils in debt to the estimated collective tune of £122 billion, we're seeing the selling off of community assets as a means of raising funds. This includes schools, care homes, boxing gyms, community centres and even an Olympic legacy equestrian centre (Lynch & Forsyth 2025). These were places where people came together to naturally meet, build friendship, develop skills and be part of a community. Not all spaces would have generated romantic partnerships (although don't underestimate the power of care homes to spark a romance or two) but their overall losses are part of a general trend of decreased community space and less natural mixing between people.

In my day, pubs and nightclubs were places where people met, flirted, got off with one another, made mistakes, had fun, had bad nights and good nights, and occasionally threw up on the pavement outside (or in a cab) but now, so many spaces have become victims of a challenging economic landscape, while also facing competition from technology-based activities. There's just more reason to stay at home than before, to choose to be up in your bedroom in isolation, rather than go out and meet people in person.

Churches have also reeled from losses in recent decades. As the son of a Baptist minister and having grown up within the culture of a large Baptist church in Sutton Coldfield town centre, most of my early romantic experiences centred around church life. However, across the UK, we've seen church numbers falling over the past 40 years, which, for the unchurched, doesn't just mean fewer people singing hymns in weekly services and taking mass in solemn silence. It means that the vibrant communities that are generally at the heart of most churches have declined too.

While there have been some recent headlines that post-Covid church numbers have been booming, particularly with young people, the evidence for a widespread and sustained revival seems patchy at best, and even those denominations that have experienced some kind of increase since the pandemic, in comparison with recent decades the overall picture is one of declining numbers.

Wherever you look, from pubs and nightclubs to churches, community spaces and youth centres, we're not naturally mixing in the way we once did. It's not that socialising and meeting new people in community settings has died out completely – and nor has dating, of course – but the way that people date today is more of a swipe, swipe, swipe, with an occasional meet-up to date, rather than a longer term, getting to know someone in a natural setting, where people meet initially through activity and shared goals. Dating has moved online and there are serious downsides for people due to this shift. More specifically, there are serious downsides for men.

Online dating: an unavoidable shift for modern daters

Tinder is the largest online dating platform and boasts more than 60 million monthly active users (Kumar 2025). In simple terms, you post your profile, and as you browse other profiles, searching for people you like, if you swipe left, you're not interested; if you swipe right, you are. If the other person also swipes right (when and if they see your profile) there's a match and correspondence is now possible. It sounds like a cattle market to me, and I appreciate that I'm old school on many things in life, but seriously, where's the natural falling in love bit? Where are the crushes that come and go as you spend lots of time with a person and realise that while you always thought they were cute, actually it's more than that, you *really* like them? And then of course, maybe you don't, but lessons have been learned.

For men, the online dating returns are quite demoralising. According to the Pew Research Center, 64 per cent of American males reported feeling insecure due to the dearth of messages they received, whereas in contrast, 54 per cent of female users said they felt overwhelmed by the sheer number of messages they received (Vogels & McClain 2023). In an early academic study of Tinder that created fake profiles and liked everyone nearby to compare how males and females fared, the male profiles matched with only about 0.6 per cent of the people they swiped on, while the female profiles matched with around 10 per cent (Graff 2017).

More recent analyses of thousands of real Tinder profiles showed the pattern has not changed. Based on Swipestats, the tool where Tinder users upload their own data, a dataset of more than 3,700 users in 2023 showed women's average match rate to be 30 per cent, while men's was 2–3 per cent. These statistics are not surprising, given that more than 70 per cent of Tinder users, in the US at least, appear to be men (Dixon 2025)!

Tinder tells of a wider story of rejection and defeat, particularly for men. I may have endured barren runs at the nightclubs in Birmingham, lean times without a girlfriend, where literally *no* females showed any romantic interest in me, and in those moments, my confidence was affected. But my only option at that time was to get back out there and be socially active, do new things, keep working at my existing hobbies and learn new ones, all of which are positive things for a man looking for romance.

Today, failure online means more time online, sitting in isolation while you search hopelessly, working against the odds on Tinder or Bumble, or drifting between Netflix binge-watching, whingeing to your mates on WhatsApp, absorbing hate-inspiring influencers or watching rubbish on Insta, TikTok and YouTube. You're sedentary in your dating habits, you're focused on the screen, you're increasingly miserable and resentful.

Lightbulb moment: Community matters

We need to see government action such as reversing both the savage cuts to youth services and the sale of community assets, so we can recreate the places to go, the things to do and access to the positive community role models we once had.

#MeToo and sextortion

In the world of post #MeToo dating, things have got messier for men. I'm glad #MeToo took off and started a global movement. Because of the awareness it created, it will be harder for future Jimmy Saviles and Mohamed Al Fayeds to carry on abusing people with no repercussions. I think the world is a safer place for children, women and girls because of #MeToo so, of course, I applaud its progress. I recognise that because of #MeToo, the world is also a safer place for most men, but within that, there may also be some unintended consequences. One of these is that good men are increasingly reserved about dating, because they fear that if they put a foot wrong out of naivety, it will be blown up and plastered all over social media.

And for anyone reading this and feeling a bit unsympathetic about a bloke getting a kicking on social media, it's worth bearing in mind that for those who have grown up with social media, it is their world. It's real life (not fake life); it's a constant and all-immersive experience. Losing your reputation on social media is no small deal and the fear of everything blowing up online is not one to be taken lightly, regardless of your gender. For many men dating today, you'll be asking yourself questions I would never have had to contemplate, such as:

- What if I take the initiative but the other person doesn't welcome it, and I get branded online as a creep or stalker? What if other people pile in with fake stories about me?
- What if things go too far physically (either within a more established relationship or as part of a one-off hook-up), but there is confusion around the issue of consent, which leads to accusations of rape or sexual assault?

When you add up the fear of getting it wrong and false accusations, together with lousy returns on Tinder and online dating in general, less natural mixing due to fewer places to mix and more people staying at home online, it's no surprise that what follows is what appears to be happening today: less intimacy, less romance, more reliance on online porn and, increasingly, AI girlfriends/boyfriends.

- A public health study of US adults released in 2020 found that a third of men aged 18–24 had not been sexually active in the previous year (Ueda et al, Mercer & Ghaznavi 2020).
- In 2023, a Pew Research Center study reported that 63 per cent of young men in America identify as single, yet back in the 1970s, 65 per cent of men by the age of 25 had already got married (King 2022)!

This is a startlingly rapid change and while more people cohabit today rather than marry, the data indicates a worrying trend: less dating, less mixing, less commitment and less confidence in initiating things. The reasons are varied and include changing aspirations, cost of living, loss of community space and so on, but another reason might be the risk of screwing up and unintentionally creating a shitstorm for yourself!

And it's not just dating that the fear of 'getting it wrong' seems to be affecting. An article published in *Fortune* research found that 60 per cent of men surveyed are afraid to mentor women at work, fearing what could happen if they meet behind closed doors or without a third-party present (Elsesser 2019). Respondents both male and female said the #MeToo movement has made it harder for men to know how to interact with women in the workplace. While it appears that false accusations of rape or sexual assault are rare (around 2–10 per cent of accusations made, depending on what research you read), the fear of the long-term impact of false accusation has left many men unsure how to interact with women (Borysenko 2020).

Sextortion is another modern phenomenon that my generation didn't have to deal with. There are two types of sextortion. The first is where people are tricked into sending intimate photographs or videos of themselves to interested dating matches online. Victims are usually groomed over time, lured in by a seemingly perfect partner who is a scammer. The scammer sends over a fake semi-nude shot of themselves and asks for one in return. The stakes keep increasing until you're sending over fully nude photos. Once the scammer has what they need (your intimate photos), the demands start arriving typically for money, with the threat that the intimate images you shared will be released to all your social media contacts, your employer, your family. It's a phenomenon that adds a dangerous risk to dating for both men and women, but one that disproportionately affects boys and men, with tragic conclusions.

In 2023 alone, the National Centre for Missing and Exploited Children in the US received 26,178 reports of financial sextortion, significantly up from the year before at 10,731 reports. We're seeing similar rises in the UK, with the Internet Watch Foundation (2024) emphasising that 90 per cent of victims of sextortion are teenage boys, and that in most of these cases it's about money. The demands never end, no matter what you pay. The data linking suicide to sextortion is patchy, but there are 20 known cases of male suicide in the US due to sextortion, with actual numbers thought to be higher (Clement-Webb 2024).

The second type of sextortion is perpetrated by bitter ex-partners who have possession of intimate photos or videos, taken while you were together and all seemed well. They're now using these to blackmail and control you. Allowing for high levels of under-reporting, overall it's estimated that 36 per cent of victims of sextortion know their sextortionist in person, with the nature of the relationship including current and former partners, family members and friends at school (Thorn 2025). It's made dating more dangerous because, if things go wrong, there may be hugely embarrassing content that the other person now has of you. Better hope they're a decent person, not too bitter and that they don't fall on hard economic times that may squeeze their previous levels of decency.

I totally get why so many young men avoid dating and watch porn instead. But if that is the reality for many men today, avoiding dating is also fraught with risk. Being single throughout life massively increases a man's risk of suicide. Bear that in mind when you think about your own wellbeing and the welfare of your sons, brothers and mates. Bear that in mind as we weigh up the direction of society on men's future outcomes.

The falling birth rate

Women are having fewer children than before and they're having them later in life. From modern contraception and women's empowerment to delayed family formation and economic barriers, if you compare UK data from 1960 to 2025, you can see just how much things have changed in a relatively short space of time, as this table shows:

	1960	**2025**
Average birth rate per woman	2.93 children	1.44 children
Average age for a women giving birth to her first child	27.8 years old	30.9 years old
Women who give birth to one child only	12 per cent	44 per cent

(Data from Beal & Smart 2024, ONS 2023 & 2024a, Hughes 2024, UK Parliament 2012.)

I'm all about women having choice. I truly believe that the work around women's equality is not complete, and I don't think feminism has gone too far. But for men, the key milestones of marriage, commitment and fatherhood are now delayed. These milestones were a catalyst for helping to mature young men, as well as bringing purpose and joy as they advanced through their twenties. With many men struggling to find their role and purpose, due to the issues explored in the previous chapter, the postponement (and increasingly, total cancellation) of such milestones simply exacerbates the sense of inadequacy, disillusion and isolation that so many men feel.

Falling birth rates are also creating another challenge for society. Loneliness affects people regardless of gender but may affect ageing men more today than ever before.

Researchers from King's College London analysed studies involving nearly 200,000 adults over the age of 50, across 21 countries, and they found that those who regularly took care of grandchildren were 60 per cent less likely to feel lonely than those who didn't (Ng 2022). The good news is that if you're an overwhelmed dad reading this and feel a bit guilty about palming the kids off onto your own parents or the in-laws, don't: you're doing them the favour! The bad news for men is you're statistically more likely to be childless in older age than a woman (Liu et al 2024), and thus less likely to have the benefits of those grandparenting duties. Therefore, your chances of experiencing loneliness in old age are greater as a man. Think of it like this: more childlessness = less grandparenting = more loneliness. It's another simple and inevitable equation that we're living with today.

When I interviewed one of the leading UK researchers on unwanted and involuntary male childlessness, Robin Hadley, for episode 26 of my podcast *Men on Show*, he made the point that 'For childless males, as you get older, whether you're living on the streets or in a block of flats, the fear of being seen as a paedophile increases.'

In a polarised world of quick judgements, social media madness and general heightened tensions within society, the paranoia of being seen as a paedophile because you're an ageing, childless male makes it even more likely that as a lonely male, you'll keep yourself to yourself and avoid certain social situations and locations, even though that approach will increase your social isolation.

Let's be clear then:

1. Older men without children or grandchildren are more likely to experience loneliness than elderly parents or elderly childless women.
2. There are more older, childless men in society than there are women.
3. As birth rates continue to fall, this issue will get worse.

Lightbulb moment: The need for compassion

We need a compassionate, intelligent and balanced approach to solving the challenges we men face today. You may feel panicked by shows like *Adolescence*, the mega-popular series on Netflix, or the stories of out-of-control young men in gangs, causing social chaos in their communities, or the rise of misogyny and toxic masculinity. These things may make you feel angry, but the root causes of why men might be struggling are complicated. Many of the causes are not the fault of the struggling person. So, as hard as it is, we have to focus on empathy and understanding if we want to change things.

The man code: why it's outdated and requires refurbishment

'Hey Andy, what's up with your face?'

I hated it when my colleagues asked me this. I hoped they wouldn't notice but they always did and it was pretty obvious. My go-to excuses to explain the bruises and cuts were shaving accidents and falling over while drunk. I wondered whether anyone would rumble me – surely a half-intelligent bloke would be unlikely to have so many 'shaving accidents' – but if they had their suspicions, they never voiced them, and had they queried my daft excuses, there's no way I could have opened up to them about what was really happening. This was the late 1990s. No one did vulnerability in the workplace back then and if you'd asked me to define domestic abuse, I would have said it was when men beat their wives or female partners, not the other way around. Even if I'd been aware of what domestic abuse was, though, I had a 'man code' to protect – a series of unwritten rules, of dos and don'ts, fashioned over time and reinforced through daily life.

The real man's man code: the dos

- Man up and be strong when times are tough. Demonstrate confidence in *all* situations.
- Keep your emotions to yourself, except for aggression and anger (which are needed to establish the upper hand).
- Never back down in an argument or fight.
- Never give up: a good man is a gritter, not a quitter.
- Make money, acquire things, maximise sexual conquests and publicise your successes, because your manliness is measured by your job, salary, house, car, holiday location, number of romantic partners and notable achievements.
- Know your shit so you're respected and adored, and if you get caught out for being wrong or unsure, don't admit it. Talk your way out of it and win.
- Provide for your family, which means hard cash, a home, a respected or flashy career, more than 'enough' material resources, holidays, gifts, the treats and the basics.
- Protect your reputation, which means fight, even if the stakes are low and the 'provocation' is trivial.
- Excel physically. Be good at sport. Maximise your physique and masculine features.

The real man's man code: the don'ts

- Don't cry or show 'weak' or 'vulnerable' emotions.
- Don't admit to mistakes or not knowing the answer.
- Don't flex or compromise: stick rigidly to your opinions.
- Don't say sorry easily or publicly: apologies are a last resort and reserved only for private conversations.
- Don't ask for help (a proper man is independent).
- Don't fail or struggle with anything anywhere.
- Don't share authority: as an adult male, you're in charge.
- Don't take interest in things that could be considered as girlie: flower arranging, midwifery, fashion design, counselling, ballet, netball. Even if they interest you, don't admit it, and find more manly pursuits.
- Don't talk about feelings. Feelings talk = Deep talk... and as blokes, we talk rubbish and focus on the banter. Feelings talk is for wimps or weirdos.

Do you recognise this man code?

If you ever wanted to make a plan for your life that ensured you failed at your relationships and lived miserably, then the stereotypical man code is a brilliant road map. You really couldn't make it up – although we did make it up: gradually and together, the man code stereotypes evolved through centuries of behaviour being conditioned to meet certain moulds. But we are not a Georgian society from the late 1700s, and just as we no longer throw our excrement out of the window or excitedly gather for a public hanging as they did back then, we need to rethink what we do with our man code today. I've heard it argued that it was men who created the man code, so it's down to men to uncreate it. But it's been made and reinforced by people over centuries and continues to be. It's up to people collectively to sort it out – and in sorting it out, we all benefit.

The good news is that we have made progress on updating the man code. The bad news is that there's still a long way to go. Let's first check out the provider stereotype and second, the idea that men should bottle up their emotions.

Real men are providers?

I know it's bonkers, but for me, the need to 'provide' in the form of housing and transport has felt like a core part of being a 'sorted' bloke. In 2009, having lost my money and assets in a divorce settlement, with no tangible job or savings left, I moved back to my parents' house, into their spare room. For the first time since renting that London flat, I was no longer able to house myself. I was lucky: without my parents, I'd have been homeless (and as a homeless single man, I would have been at the very bottom of the council's priority list). But as lucky as I was to have such awesome parents who could house me, rent free and in a nice house, the inability to stand on my own feet made me feel inadequate, powerless and emasculated. I couldn't get beyond thinking that a real man would be able to fend for himself and provide materially, and anything less was a reflection of my stupidity and weakness. It may sound daft, but I was certainly not alone in my thinking about men and their responsibility to provide.

As part of the 'State of American Men 2025' report, 86 per cent of men surveyed chose 'providing for my family' as the top trait that defined true manhood. They didn't choose virility, bicep measurements, penile size or number of sexual adventures or conquests; they chose 'providing for my family' – and most women surveyed (77 per cent) concurred with this view of man as provider (Equimundo 2025).

In a 2024 study of 3,000 young adults between the ages of 18 and 24 in the UK, 70 per cent of Gen Z men believed that men should be the breadwinner in the family, with 60 per cent saying that men would feel emasculated if their female partners earned more (Starling Bank 2024). Bearing in mind the economic and social challenges that many of us are facing today, this stereotype fuels men's sense of inadequacy and shame when we can't measure up. At the same time, and to compound the experiences for men at the lower economic end of society, women are more independent today than before, so they can be choosier over whom they settle down with and when.

According to research from the Office for National Statistics and the House of Commons Library (both 2025), the number of employed women in the UK has significantly increased since the 1970s, and at the same time, the number of employed men has dropped (almost as significantly as the growth in the number of employed women). For example, in the UK, the percentage of working-age women who are employed has grown from 52 per cent in the 1970s to 72 per cent in the 2020s, while the number of employed men of working age in the UK has dropped from 92 per cent to 78 per cent within the same timescale. Again, I applaud the gains made by women in the working environment. It's the kind of progress women have been struggling to achieve for decades. But yet, as women have been progressing, the old stereotype of man as provider hasn't faded, either in the minds of men or of women.

Maybe the reason it hasn't faded is because if you're a man with resources, you'll genuinely find it easier to secure a romantic partner who is happy to settle down with you. So the stereotype endures because while the world has changed on the one hand (with female emancipation and increased participation levels in the job market), on the other hand it hasn't changed because men who can provide rule OK in the reproduction and fatherhood stakes.

Given this is a provocative statement, let's head to Norway to test it out. Using Norwegian registry data on all births since 1967, male childlessness was found to be as high as 72 per cent among the lowest 5 per cent of earners, but only 11 per cent among the highest earners, and this is a gap that has significantly widened in the past 30 years. So, let's be clear, if you're financially disadvantaged as a man – in Norway at least – then your chances of becoming a father are significantly reduced, compared with those of a high earner (Bratsberg et al 2021). And long term? As we've just explored, you're likely to be lonelier in old age with no grandparenting duties and as an elderly childless male, you may have the added stigma of being seen as a paedophile.

The man as provider stereotype arguably holds firm because there's some truth in it when it comes to selection and reproduction. But after years of deindustrialisation, a housing crisis and austerity, there are very large numbers of men who just can't provide in the way their grandfathers did, and that inability to provide is both isolating and heartbreaking. It's not their fault. It's not your fault. Society has rapidly changed, but much of the outdated man code hasn't.

Real men don't cry?

I like to call out success when I see it and there is an area of change that should inspire us all. To me, this one change demonstrates that ancient stereotypes can be unpicked and recycled. It's the notion that proper men don't cry. Growing up, I definitely knew that I shouldn't cry in public, that if I was seen to cry as a man, it would say something about my lack of manliness, so best to cry alone quietly, keep it to myself and not talk about it. Brave men don't cry!

I remember the 1990 football World Cup, and the England men's team's performance in it, so vividly. We came close to ending the national pain. We scraped and scrapped our way to the semi-finals. England did not play pretty football (aside from a sublime David Platt goal against Belgium), but one player stood out: Paul Gascoigne, one of the finest English players of all time, and who has had a quite remarkable career given his mental health challenges. When England lost on penalties in the semi-finals, Gascoigne shed tears, and his tears were a media sensation: they were headline news. It was so 'unusual' that Walker's Crisps even created an advertising campaign out of his tearful moment. It stood out because this stuff just didn't happen. But wind the clock forward to today, and when elite male sports stars cry – out of either joy or sadness, or simply the scale of the occasion – there's no fuss and it all feels quite normal.

Society, in the UK and beyond, has made some progress on this particular stereotype, but aside from 'some' progress on this one angle, broadly speaking, while the world has dramatically changed, the stereotypical man code has not kept up. I will return to the man code and what to do about it in the final chapter of this book.

We've been on a journey to uncover some of the more complex issues behind why men are struggling – and I've not even discussed negative media messaging, political laziness, technology and the testosterone crisis, each of which are explored in the next chapters. But hopefully what you can already see is that there is no one answer or magic solution, that men struggle for complex reasons rather than being inherently toxic as men. And if you're a struggling bloke feeling lost in the world, I hope you can see that it's not your fault – many of the causes are no one's fault. But they have happened.

We need strong men to boldly challenge the man code stereotypes, and for the rest of us to tell their stories, putting a spotlight on their work. One of my podcast guests particularly stands out and his story is a fitting way to close this chapter.

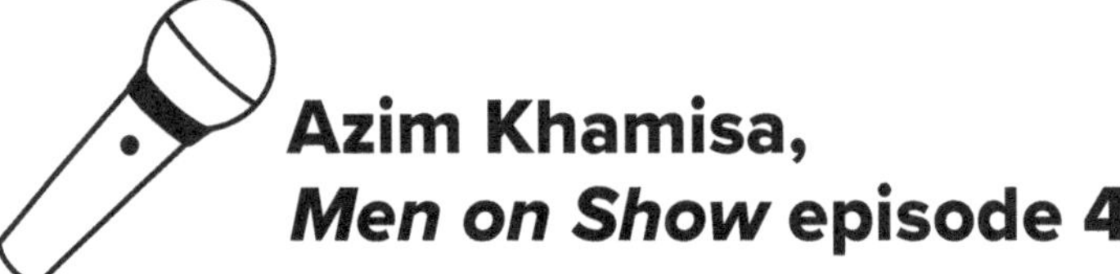

Azim Khamisa, *Men on Show* episode 4

> Azim's only son, Tariq, was murdered while delivering pizza. He was lured to a bogus address and robbed, then shot by a 14-year-old called Tony. Amid the grief and unbearable horror, Azim forgave Tony, understanding that there were two victims at the scene: Tariq and Tony. They're both victims of American gun culture. Azim then mentored Tony and went on to campaign for his release. He also completed the most emotionally charged TED talk I've ever seen, with Tony's grandfather. Azim has gone on to create a forgiveness project which has been taken up around the world.

Strong male superheroes: they do exist, although they don't all wear capes, and they may not have huge biceps and pecs. They're not in hiding; they're out there tirelessly serving like Azim Khamisa – it's just that their stories are often missed by the media, who need to sell clicks and newspapers, which means focusing on sex, gossip and horror, rather than wonderful men who make the world a better place. Their stories are missed because when it comes to the media, negativity about men is a much better seller than positivity, as we're about to find out in the next chapter.

4 Men are not toxic – but the narrative about men is

> "How do we stop this kid becoming a monster?"
>
> Article from *The West Australian*, reported on Sky News Australia (Panahi 2023)

This was the headline in the Australian press in the autumn of 2023. The question was accompanied by a photo of an innocent-looking 11- to 12-year-old boy and the tagline read: 'Call for Domestic Violence lessons at all schools to address menace of toxic masculinity.' What are we supposed to make of this headline? How would my own 12-year-old son feel if he read this?

What about an impressionable male teenager, online for hour after hour in isolation? What if he had two working parents who he barely connects with, no siblings at home and a vague interest in Andrew Tate? How would this headline impact his thinking?

I don't recall this general narrative growing up. I was not made to feel that in getting sweatier, hairier, girl-focused, drunker on occasions, a bit lippier and more self-focused, I was somehow becoming a monstrous man, toxic male and all-round misogynist. Nor do I recall a divisive female/male gender war or messaging around 'girl power' and 'the future is female'. Had I absorbed this kind of message, it might have made me resentful towards authority and women in general. It might have encouraged me to behave according to the narrative, simply out of a 'screw-you' and bloody-minded mentality.

In this chapter, I'm going to examine how messaging in the media is currently skewed against men and why that is damaging for us. I'll also put a spotlight on how governments have steered clear of creating strategy and spending resources on exclusively male causes. These things matter because the approach taken by media and government sets the tone for how society then thinks and talks about that topic. With better awareness, you'll be equipped to spot the negative bias when it occurs, so we can all call it out, as well as push our politicians for change, something that will help the current and next generation of men – which is good news for everyone.

In March 2025, *The Independent* newspaper published an article with a headline strikingly similar to that in Australia: 'Schools to run anti-misogyny classes for boys in bid to tackle toxic masculinity.'

The article explains how in the light of the popular Netflix series, *Adolescence*, school children in the UK are set to be given lessons in how to tackle misogyny and toxic masculinity, amid the rise of influencers such as Andrew Tate. If I'd been reading this article as a male teenager, Tate would immediately have become far more appealing to me than he might otherwise have been. As a teen, anything that might horrify responsible adults immediately feels cool, and for a generation of young men who feel that their challenges are ignored, and that they're unfairly blamed for the issues in the world, of course they're going to look to Tate as an intriguing, rogue outlaw.

From *The Independent* to one of my most hated British newspapers, *The Daily Moan* (it's official name: *The Daily*

Mail). This article is from 2025: 'Is your son a ticking timebomb? From not letting you see his phone, to being rude to his mother, expert reveals signs to watch out for.'

I suspect there may be a few mums and dads reading this, thinking of their daughters who are equally rude to them and obstruct any sense of parental oversight or authority when it comes to the phone and social media. This isn't just a boy problem, and the article is typical fearmongering about males, hoping to tap into parents' insecurities with an alarming message that goes something like this:

'That lovely fella who you know and love as your son... you know, the one with curly locks, charming smile and nice attitude: you knew him in the womb, drooled over the scan photos and he's made your heart melt for years with his warmth and character, but watch out, he's fast growing up and it's only a matter of time until he turns into a monstrous man.'

In an article posted by the American Institute for Boys and Men in 2024, Catherine Carr, an award-winning documentary-maker, presenter and reporter, interviewed young men about the negative male-focused language they hear and how it impacts them. They complained about regularly hearing the 'kill all men' phrase and felt mystified by it. They didn't understand why men were considered bad and understandably felt a sense of shame for being male.

Framing men, boys and masculinity as the problem and insinuating that poor male behaviour is down to rotten male genes has contributed to the issues many men face today, affecting how we feel about our worth, particularly at a period in history when many of us are struggling to grasp our purpose and role in society (for reasons I've examined in Chapters 2 and 3).

In a survey of 4,000 men (2,000 from Germany and 2,000 from the UK), it was found that men who perceived their own gender positively were more likely to experience good mental health, whereas those who viewed their gender negatively (ie toxic males, out-of-control misogynists, lazy bystanders) had worse mental health (Dolan 2023). So, maybe it's not surprising that so many of us feel so lousy about ourselves when the general narrative about men and toxic masculinity has become quite normal:

- Two blokes scrapping in a pub? It's toxic masculinity!
- Men who won't go to the doctor when they have symptoms? It's toxic masculinity!
- Men who struggle to articulate their feelings, so they bottle it up? It's toxic masculinity!

As a popular buzzword today, 'toxic masculinity' is used to explain a sweeping range of 'typical' male behaviour. But a better starting point for constructive conversation would be to ditch the phrase and accept that some people have destructive tendencies towards self and others, and these are usually due to complex reasons.

Labelling male struggles as 'toxic masculinity' simply risks a lazy approach to analysing what's really going on and diagnosing way too early. If a man is struggling, it may have a lot to do with poverty, unemployment, an empathy gap, societal expectations, poor mental health, poor physical health or his ACEs (adverse childhood experiences, such as bereavement, poverty, parental separation, domestic abuse, bullying, each of which can have a profound long-term effect on people, stretching into adulthood and old age).

Keith Fraser was my third podcast guest, a former superintendent and chief inspector in the West Midlands Police with expertise on gang and youth violence. On the podcast, he describes why he's not a fan of the toxic masculinity label for two specific reasons:

'It can encourage men to stick to that kind of culture and reinforce the stereotype. It can also cause others to fear men and that's awful. Neither of these outcomes are positive.'

Lightbulb moment: Inspiration in place of toxicity

> 'Toxic masculinity' is both lazy and toxic language. Let's call it out and find more compassionate, inspirational rhetoric to engage the men and boys in our lives.

Deadbeat dads, perpetrators and predators

There are other powerful yet negative narratives about men that shape how we think about ourselves, including the notion of men as useless, deadbeat dads, in need of man-keeping (so therefore it's better we're treated as misbehaving children rather than rational adults).

The Guardian posted an article in 2024 about dads who take paternity leave when their children are born so Mum can go back to work (Dizik 2024). Within the article, there were no reflections from those dads working tirelessly to support Mum or from family units where Mum is gutted to be back at work because she desperately wants to be at home with the baby, but it's just that she is the bigger earner and as a couple they can't afford for her to be at home. Instead, the article focused on bashing dads for taking liberties when on paternity leave, palming the kids off so they can spend time in the gym, grabbing 'me time' as typically selfish males are prone to doing. The overriding sentiment of the article is 'poor Mum'! She is now doubly screwed because she still has the housework to do when she gets home from work. The article includes some choice snippets, so let's analyse them and unpick some of the gender biases:

> 'Men can pick to take it when it's convenient for them or when it will benefit them the most. Some even take the time off in a way that won't impact their annual bonus.'

(Maybe, for these men, their annual bonus really matters because they want to provide for their family unit? Maybe the annual bonus is not his beer money or ticket for the lads' skiing holiday. Maybe securing the bonus enables mum to go back to work as late as possible because she wants maximum time with the baby.)

> 'Even for fathers who are the main caretakers during their leave, it's the mothers who continue to bear the brunt of developmental milestones or who get calls from the paediatrician's office, even when the father is listed first...'

(This is a people problem and it's common. Even when dads are listed as the first point of contact at school for the kids, it's often Mum who is called. But that's not Dad's fault and statistically, given that there are far more female staff in schools than male staff, it's more likely to be females making the decision to call Mum rather than Dad.)

> 'For fathers who do take paternity leave to pursue hobbies or get fit, it can also fall in line with their vision of becoming a complete father, thinking: "I'm going to do this for myself..."'

(Seriously, what proportion of dads who take paternity leave do so in order to 'pursue a hobby' as their primary reason? If it's genuinely a 'thing', show me the research! Until then, this is wittering and musings. It's not serious journalism.)

> 'On the other hand, mothers have so much of the physical and mental stuff to contend with during their leave that there is not time for them to even consider themselves holistically.'

(Parenting overwhelm is a common problem for mums *and* dads, as I'll explore in the chapter on fatherhood.)

In Jim Macnamara's book, *Media and Male Identity: The making and remaking of men* (2006), he drew on hundreds of articles and reports from 650 newspapers, more than 100 magazines and more than 330 hours of TV, across multiple countries. Macnamara found that in more than 80 per cent of articles, men were portrayed negatively: as villains, perpetrators, aggressors, workaholics, deadbeat dads, perverts and philanderers. While his work is increasingly dated (the original findings are from 20 years ago), if the same research were carried out today, it's fair to suggest that the 80 per cent figure is unlikely to have dropped.

In fact, in research from 2025, Professor Lara Wood from Abertay University analysed more than 1,900 animal characters from children's animated movies, focusing on the gender of predators and prey. Even when accounting for a much higher number of male characters within the movies she studied, 85 per cent of predator characters were male, with most female characters as prey. Yet in the animal kingdom, a predator animal is no more likely to be male than female.

Through the media and from the earliest ages, our children are fed traditional, negative stereotypes about males, and this continues into adulthood. It's no wonder so many of us men feel lost, disillusioned and depressed. It's hardly much of a rallying cry to inspire us. Some might argue that the negative media messaging about men is a fair reflection of where we are today in society: just look at all the awful men out there doing terrible things, and if men want the messaging to change, then we need to change first. But the reality is that most men are amazing, and there is no shortage of everyday male superheroes in society today; it's just that they rarely wear capes, and their stories go untold.

Male heroes under the radar

The prestigious Carnegie Medal for bravery has quite exacting standards – if you ever wanted one for your CV. These standards include:

- The rescuer must be a civilian who knowingly and voluntarily risks his or her own life to an extraordinary degree.
- The rescuer must have rescued or attempted the rescue of another person.
- The act of rescue must be one in which no full measure of responsibility exists between the rescuer and the rescued (it's expected that a parent would risk their own life to rescue their child from a riptide, but jumping to the aid of someone else's child is a different matter).
- There must be conclusive evidence to support the threat to the victim's life, the risk undertaken by the rescuer, the rescuer's degree of responsibility and the act's occurrence (these are not awarded on the basis of hearsay).

Of the 10,000 recipients of the medal since 1904, 90 per cent are male, with 25 per cent of medals being awarded posthumously (Carnegie Hero Fund). But could you name any of the stories or heroes? I know I couldn't. So, what happened to those stories? And why aren't they retold again and again? Why are they not part of global folklore?

Negativity, gossip, sex, infidelity, getting rich quick, misbehaving people, toxic men – these are bestsellers, but uplifting stories about everyday male heroes generally aren't. Even when an event involving a male hero is so massive that it makes it into the global media, the maleness of the heroes is downplayed or just not mentioned and you can forget any trending hashtags, such as: #menrockingit #supermen #manpower or #thesemendo.

Instead, let's stick to the facts. Let's not sensationalise, for example, the fact that in July 2018, a group of selfless, humble, middle-aged men from the UK headed out to Thailand at enormous personal risk, not because they had to, but because they felt compelled to do the right thing, to pull off a seemingly impossible rescue of 12 teenage boys and their coach trapped deep inside a flooded cave complex with water levels rising. A rescue that, frankly, no one else in the world could have achieved.

Thai Navy Seals had attempted to find the boys, deep inside the flooded caves, but the extreme cave conditions were beyond their expertise and beyond the expertise of the other experts who had assembled in Thailand. The job fell to Rick Stanton, John Volanthen and Robert Harper, highly experienced and respected cave divers, to plan, lead and execute the rescue, supported by an additional team of British male cave divers – and of course the wider support onsite of hundreds of local and international volunteers – to pull off a miracle.

They got everyone out in the nick of time, drawing on courage, selflessness, extraordinary skill, extensive experience and meticulous planning. There was plenty of celebration around the world, plenty of gratitude, yet nothing was made of the all-male nature of that diving team. What a shame that among the messaging around toxic masculinity, our media aren't also taking the opportunity to put a spotlight on the actions of amazing men, celebrating their achievements to inspire the next and current generation of men in positive ways.

On my podcast *Men on Show*, there is story after story of everyday male heroes. Two fellas out of the many stand out to me.

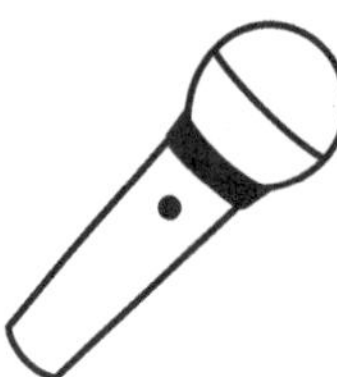

Ricky Nuttall, *Men on Show* episode 30

Ricky Nuttall is a former firefighter and one of the first respondents at the Grenfell Tower disaster, the tragic and preventable inferno that broke out in the high-rise, 24-storey tower block of flats in London on 14 June 2017. It tragically claimed the lives of 72 people. Ricky put his life on the line, pushing his equipment well beyond safety protocols, braving heat of 550°C on the 15th floor – a heat that was burning him even under all his protection gear – running his air tank to the absolute end, barely making it out (even though he is a father whose son was three at the time). Like so many firefighters that night, not only were they heroes in that inferno, they then went back following the fire to do a job that, frankly, no one in their right mind would want to do, but a job that had to be done nonetheless: recover the charred bodies of the people they'd been unable to rescue only a few nights before.

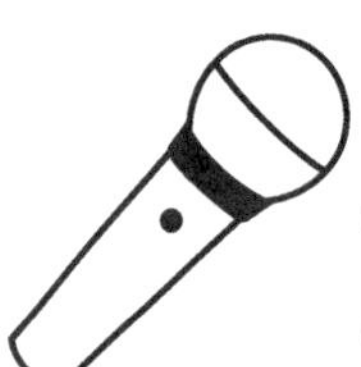

Adam Smith: *Men on Show* episode 10

Adam Smith grew up in a hugely dysfunctional home and was eventually sectioned, imprisoned and came close to dying by suicide. But in the years that followed, he went on to found the multi-award-winning global initiative the Real Junk Food Project (TRJFP). This revolutionised the disposal of avoidable food waste into landfill, operating with the memorable tagline 'Feed bellies, not bins'. The movement was pivotal in changing people's attitude towards food waste, spearheading a global food movement.

Ricky Nuttall and Adam Smith: just two of many examples I could share from my podcast alone. The male heroes are out there. In fact, if you really start thinking about the men you know and what they do, you'll realise they're everywhere. And we don't just have male heroes today. They've always been there in society. 'Women and children first' – do you know where that protocol came from? It's the Birkenhead drill, whose origins lie in a legendary act of discipline and self-sacrifice by British soldiers during the sinking of HMS *Birkenhead* in 1852. There weren't enough lifeboats for the 643 people on board (476 of whom were soldiers), so the soldiers stood in formation on deck, allowing women and children to be evacuated first. Most of the soldiers either drowned or were taken by sharks.

We just don't hear enough about amazing men. So on the one hand, we have negative messaging about men and boys – which stretches beyond the media and into our communities and political circles – and on the other hand, we are reluctant to celebrate the everyday male heroes in the world, of which there are plenty and always have been. When you throw into the mix an empathy gap, it's no wonder that so many of us men feel so rotten about ourselves.

Lightbulb moment: Celebrate male excellence

I'm all for celebrating female achievement *and* I hope we can be as excited by male achievement too. I want my sons' achievements to be celebrated as much as my daughters'. When we think about the next generation of young men, wouldn't you want them to have easy access to countless, real-life stories of everyday male heroes? Wouldn't you want the existing generation of men to be inspired by positive male heroes like the guys from my podcast, rather than Tate, the Liver King (see the next chapter, on technology, if you haven't yet heard of him) and other online charlatans?

The empathy gap

In a recent and large-scale study of 35,000 people in the US, which examined their attitudes towards men and women, researchers found that people in general are more accepting of men suffering than women. It also found that when men have fallen behind, people are more likely to see this as due to a lack of effort, whereas for women, it's more likely to be seen as the result of systemic failure (ie not their personal fault). Or if men are in poor health, it's due to their behavioural issues rather than external factors (Cappelen et al 2025).

We're lacking our sense of empathy for half the human population and if we're serious about creating a more cohesive society, we need to rediscover it. The research from the US is not an isolated piece of work. In November 2024, researchers Maja Graso and Tania Reynolds published an article that recounted wide-ranging studies and experiments illustrating that people were more sympathetic towards women than men, particularly women of childbearing age. In a variety of experiments, it was found that:

- people are more prepared to sacrifice men than women
- people experienced more pity when exposed to photographs of women in pain than men in pain
- people were less willing to support interventions that caused collateral harm to women than those that might cause identical harm to men.

Reynolds and Graso pointed to the evolutionary pressures of growing the human race as a subconscious reason for these dynamics, whereby, to ensure the survival of any species, you'd be better off with plenty of females and fewer males, rather than vice versa. Over time, this understanding has evolved into what we have today: an instinctive protection of women, girls and male children, and a lack of concern for male suffering.

In 2016, *Time* magazine published an article in relation to the Boko Haram kidnappings several years before. We should of course be outraged about the kidnapping of more than 250 girls by this extremist group, but in the previous three years, they'd also kidnapped more than 10,000 boys, something that received no global media spotlight. The *Time* article draws on comments made by former US Secretary of State Hillary Clinton: 'My heart aches for the hundreds of boys and girls who have been kidnapped by Boko Haram over the years.'

Clinton goes on to refer to their abduction as 'a stark reminder of the work we must do to advance equality for women and girls'.

In the wider article, other than the one comment about her heart aching for boys as well as girls, the entire focus is about the girls and that the kidnapping is a clear example of the need to do more global work for women and girls. There is no mention of missing boys, or their predicament as kidnapped boys, or the sheer number of male victims in comparison with the female victims.

The empathy gap creates a general impression that men and boys are disposable, that their suffering is nothing to get worked up about. But we are not disposable. My sons are not disposable. My dad is not disposable. You are not disposable. Our challenges and suffering are as worthy of attention as those of the women and girls we love.

Male = perpetrator, female = victim

Recently, the findings of a startling study from Australia were made public. Drawing on the answers from 26,000 men, one in three men surveyed admitted to using 'partner violence' in their lifetime. Just in case you missed that, let me spell it out: one in three Australian men admits to being guilty of domestic violence at some point in his life or on an ongoing basis. Carried out by the Australian Institute of Family Studies and drawing on a decent sample size, the findings understandably caused quite a stir in Australia and beyond, being reported in the UK's *Guardian* in June 2025 with the following headline: 'One in three Australian men has reported committing domestic violence, world-first research has found.' (Shepherd 2025)

ABC News in Australia said the research makes a key contribution to ending family and domestic violence in Australia and I must admit, when I first saw the headline, I felt initially angry towards Australian men.

- What's going on in Australia?
- Why are their men like that?
- Is it the same here in the UK, but just hidden?

But wait just a moment. Let's look at the small print before we feel too mad at Australian men. Later in the article, there is a troubling yet understated paragraph, where the *Guardian* slips into the article the following words: 'The definition of intimate partner violence includes emotional as well as physical abuse'. Respondents were invited to answer "yes" or "no" to the following two questions:

- Have you ever behaved in a manner that has made a partner feel frightened or anxious? (emotional-type abuse)
- Have you ever hit, slapped, kicked or otherwise physically hurt a partner when you were angry? (physical violence)'

The reality is that only 9 per cent of those 26,000 men surveyed answered 'yes' to the second question, with 35 per cent answering 'yes' to the first question.

Do you see the issue?

I'm a gentle man, easy-going and more likely to lose my temper with a malfunctioning object than a person, but have I *ever* behaved in a manner that has made my wife today feel frightened or anxious?

Of course I have – who hasn't?

What wife or husband has never behaved in a way that might make their spouse feel anxious? As a question it's either laughably absurd or written to catch men out in order to create some juicy headlines. Let me put it this way: imagine I dated someone who struggled with anxiety. How would I ensure I never made her feel anxious? It wouldn't be possible. If I had been part of that survey, I would have had to answer 'yes' to the first question, so by definition, I'm guilty of partner violence too!

The correct media headlines therefore are these:

- Around one in ten Australian men (just under 9 per cent) has admitted to using physical violence against a partner in their lifetime.
- 35 per cent of Australian men admitted to having at one point or another made their partner feel frightened or anxious for whatever reason.

- Over half of those surveyed were lying because it's not possible to truthfully answer 'no' to the first question. (Have you ever behaved in a manner that has made a partner feel frightened or anxious?)

There is another glaring problem with this research. Why were women not also surveyed with the same questions about their behaviour towards their partners? It's what's known as 'gamma bias', a term coined by psychologists Dr John Barry and Martin Seager and used to describe how male suffering is downplayed, male privilege is exaggerated and male wrongdoing is emphasised, while the opposite often happens with women.

The 'one in three Australian men' headline is just one example of how the media reports on issues relating to men and women. You can see a similar dynamic in the UK, where the common narrative in the media and parliament about domestic violence is that the overwhelming majority of victims of domestic abuse are women, and the overwhelming majority of perpetrators are men. But according to the Crime Survey for England and Wales, in the year ending 25 March 2025, it's estimated that 2.2 million females and 1.5 million males, aged 16 years and over, experienced domestic abuse in the last year (ONS 2025b). So certainly the greater proportion of victims are female according to data, but the perception of an 'overwhelming majority' is misleading.

From domestic abuse to safeguarding, there is a bias that sees men as potential perpetrators, and this is damaging for many men.

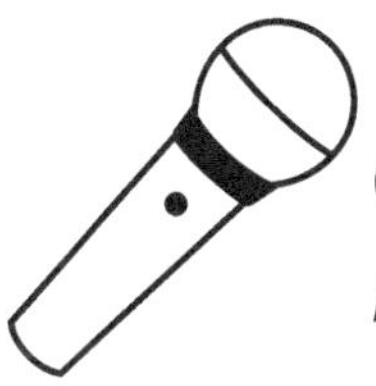

Charlie Bethel, *Men on Show*, episode 16

Charlie Bethel is the former CEO of Men's Sheds Association. With more than 1,000 sheds in the UK, it's mostly men who come together to make things, renovate things and form a community. When I asked him about the challenges his organisation faces, he referred to the bias against men, citing one example where the association had sought permission to create a shed in a community space, but they'd been refused by the council because the space was opposite a school. As the shed would be likely to engage mostly men, the initiative was seen by the council as a safeguarding risk. While the group did not fight the decision, some of the men involved in trying to secure permission at that site were grandfathers of the children of the school in question and spoke of their distress at the stance taken by the council.

So, you may be wondering: if the narrative about men is not generally positive, and there's an empathy gap, if male heroes go under the radar and men are generally seen as perpetrators with women as victims, does this mix really impact how men feel about themselves? For me, as a privileged, middle-class man, it's more of an irritation, but for less privileged men and for those who are struggling, it's offensive and simply isolates them in their suffering.

- Why would you ask for help if you suspect people won't take your suffering seriously?
- Why would you ask for help if the default position is

to see you as the more likely perpetrator due to your gender?

- Why would you feel positive about yourself if you're part of a species (male) which is disposable, not worthy of celebration and the cause of most of the world's problems?

Aside from how this mix may affect us as men, it also impacts how politicians think about us.

Lightbulb moment: Equal empathy

We're more likely to have more empathy for women than men because we've been conditioned that way, so let's be mindful of this when we see newspaper headlines about one in three Australian men admitting to domestic violence. Let's stand back to assess the quality of the research before forming our conclusions about Australian men – that would be a good starting point.

Once we're aware of the empathy gap, we're more likely to see the double standards at play in the world of employment, where, for example, underrepresentation of women in male-dominated fields such as engineering is often attributed to discrimination and addressed through intervention, but we don't question men's underrepresentation in female-dominated fields such as nursing, nor do we argue that there should be intervention to remedy it. Intervention usually costs money.

Political laziness in the UK

Misogyny v misandry

Between 2018 and 2022, moves were made by mostly Labour and Liberal Democrat MPs to make misogyny a formal hate crime in the UK. They argued that doing so would send a clear signal of intent for protecting women and girls, as well as promoting cultural change and aiding the police in their recording of misogynistic crime. Ultimately, the bill was rejected by mostly Conservative MPs, who cited concerns about overburdening police, not addressing root causes of misogyny and potentially creating a confusing overlap with existing laws on harassment, domestic abuse and rape.

What no one raised at the time or has done since (other than me banging my drum) was a very simple point: that had misogyny become a formal hate crime, then rhetoric or behaviour that might be perceived as misogynistic in nature would be illegal and risk a conviction, while hateful behaviour or rhetoric towards men (misandry) would simply be an unwanted nuisance, but nothing to trouble the police with and certainly not warranting a conviction.

Let's unpack this a bit more with the following hypothetical situation. Imagine the initiative to make misogyny a formal hate crime made it through Parliament and had been written into law. No doubt women's groups would have been celebrating this as a step forward.

Then, one day in a sixth-form college in the UK, there follows a one-off and verbal tirade from an 18-year-old male student towards another 18-year-old female student. His verbal outburst was both hateful and misogynistic in nature (thus breaking the law) but the evidence also showed that the female student had preceded his tirade with comments about males that were entirely hateful towards men (misandrist).

Technically, he would be prosecuted in this scenario, but she wouldn't.

- How might that have been received by the young men at that school?
- How would the teachers square that with their students if challenged?
- If you're a father of a son reading this (or a mother), imagine if your son was the male student in question in this scenario: would you think that's fair enough?

Either misogyny and misandry go through together as hate crimes, and with careful thought about how to police them, or neither is a hate crime. You can't have one as a hate crime and the other not. The empathy gap: it not only plays out in the way we think about men and women in our communities, it plays out at Parliament and came quite close to creating legislation which would have added to the gender division by targeting hateful men, but not hateful women.

We have a VAWG and we need a VAMB

In a former relationship, I was the victim of domestic violence and as a male victim of violence whose perpetrator was female, in the eyes of the law, I was a victim of violence against women and girls.

Confused?

You should be. I'm still a bit confused by it.

In 2010, a government Strategy to Tackle Violence against Women and Girls was initiated. It's commonly referred to as VAWG. At the same time, a strategy to tackle violence against men and boys was... hmm... well... this is a bit awkward... it wasn't thought about or discussed, so there isn't one!

Let me spell this out. There is no equivalent Violence against Men and Boys strategy (VAMB), so all initiatives, discourse, debate and data for male victims of violence are swept into VAWG strategy. You may have picked up on statements in the press such as 'Violence against women and girls is an epidemic', but what is closer to the truth is

'Violence against people is an epidemic' – because included in the data for violence against women and girls is the data for male victims too.

I like to steer clear of conspiracy theories but sometimes situations crop up where there just doesn't seem to be a logical reason for why something happened in the way it did, and the lack of a VAMB is one of those situations. Successive Victims Commissioners, such as Dame Vera Baird and the late Baroness Newlove, have been at pains to lobby for a separate VAMB strategy, but there is still no government commitment.

Duncan Craig (OBE), my 42nd podcast guest on *Men on Show*, was at the heart of the action when the VAWG strategy was first announced. He contributed towards the pivotal government-commissioned review by Baroness Vivien Stern back in 2006 and 2007. I asked him on the podcast why no VAMB was created when VAWG was. He was there on the ground at the time: he should know. I was hopeful for a new angle on the topic that would make some sense of it. He explained that as the VAWG strategy was being created, he was regularly involved in Home Office and NHS meetings and for any conspiracy theorists out there, prepare to be disappointed: he says there was no deliberate plan to squash a strategy for men and boys.

VAWG just happened and VAMB didn't. Men and boys weren't mentioned or really thought about. Maybe it was a Birkenhead drill moment (women and children/girls first) or simply a reflection of the unconscious empathy gap. But as Duncan Craig emphasises, the point of creating a separate VAMB strategy today is that it could create focus on preventing suicide and knife crime, for example – both of which disproportionately affect men and boys as victims. It would make a lot of sense, but we're still waiting... and waiting... and waiting...

Where's our minister for men?

Alongside a lack of a VAMB, we don't have a minister for men either – yet. The role of minister for women and girls was created in 1997 under the Tony Blair government, its purpose to address the inequalities that disproportionately affect women. The minister for women is a hugely important role, leading government strategy for gender equality, promoting women's representation in public life, advocating for improvements for women's health and wellbeing, and representing the UK internationally at summits and forums focused on women's rights. The role is so pivotal that there have been calls for it to become a standalone role which sits at the heart of the cabinet.

For more than 25 years, we've had a minister for women active within Parliament, but not once in that time have we had a minister for men. And just in case you wondered if anyone has ever asked for one, they most definitely have. But the idea is yet to be taken forward and, most recently at the time of writing, it was entirely dismissed by UK prime minister Sir Kier Starmer. The common objections I hear when this proposal is discussed are:

- Just because women have a minister, it doesn't mean that men need one or should have one.
- This is simply 'whataboutery' from men, who need to get over themselves.
- There aren't the resources for one and if there was a bit of spare cash in the public coffers, the money would be best spent elsewhere.

The minister for men could mirror the work of the minister for women, addressing male-specific issues while not detracting from women's equality work. And given the issues that I examined in Chapter 1 (from loneliness to life expectancy, suicide, prison, education and homelessness), there are plenty of pressing issues that affect men. A central role in Parliament could help join the dots, connect often fragmented outputs from organisations working with men and advocate for change. It's less about 'whataboutery' and more about impact, moral courage and common sense. To not have a minister for men sends this clear message:

Women are still struggling (hence the minister for women) but men are largely not, so if you're a man and you're struggling, it's probably your fault, so try a bit harder.

The lack of political willpower sets the tone of the wider conversation around men's issues, so it's no wonder that many men feel unsupported, forgotten and disillusioned by mainstream government, which leaves them exposed to manipulation from extremist political voices and, practically speaking, it leaves many struggling men without support.

Signs of change on both sides of the ocean

The good news is that things are changing for the better. Increasingly, governments are waking up to the male crisis and embracing the notion that we can advocate for men and women at the same time. As referenced in Chapter 1, Wes Streeting, Secretary of State for Health and Social Care, announced the UK's Men's Health Strategy in November 2025. Broadly welcomed by men's campaigners on all sides of the political spectrum, this is an important step forward – one that follows on the heels of the creation of a Women's Health Strategy in 2022, which hopefully provides a political foundation for creating a separate strategy to tackle violence against men and boys (VAMB) and a minister for men.

In his written ministerial foreword, which starts the strategy, Streeting says: 'It can be tough to be a man in today's society... Society has been slow to wake up to the fact that a lot of men and boys are really struggling and I am grateful to all those who have picked up this agenda and forced it into the mainstream... this strategy is not just a plan, it is a call to action: to create a society where men and boys are supported to live longer, healthier and happier lives; where stigma is replaced by understanding; and where every man knows that his health matters.'

And there have been promising signs from across the ocean, too. On the *IMO* podcast, hosted by Michelle Obama and Craig Robinson, former US president Barack Obama explored the themes of fatherhood and masculinity. He was unequivocal in his summing-up of the handling of men's issues by the political left and liberals to date:

'Democrats, progressive parents, enlightened ones, we've made that mistake sometimes in terms of our rhetoric, where it's like we're constantly talking about what's wrong with the boys instead of what's right with them. We rightly have tried to invest in girls to make sure that there's a level playing field and they're not barred from opportunities. But we haven't been as willing to be intentional about investing in the boys, and that's been a mistake.'

Negative media messaging and political laziness are contributory factors to the issues men face today. Things are slowly changing for the better but there is much to do.

Lightbulb moment: Supporting men is a win–win

Barack Obama is right. I'm hugely encouraged that such a prominent global figure has spoken up, which is why his words have closed off this chapter. Supporting men, celebrating men and advocating for their welfare is a step in the right direction for everyone. It's a win–win, *not* a win for men and a loss for women.

5 Men and technology

Technology is a beautiful thing: it's changed our lives beyond recognition and created a world that would have been unimaginable only 100 years ago. But as useful and convenient as technology is, it carries painful side effects, too. From porn to gambling, gossip and human envy, the online world has exacerbated the negative impact of these vices – vices that always existed in society, but today are in infinite supply, 24/7.

We don't struggle with online addictions because we're weak or naïve. We struggle with them because we're human and every element of our online world has been built with two key aims:

1. retain the attention of the user so they don't log off or move to another platform

2. ensure that when they do log off (due to needing to eat or go to the loo), they come straight back for more.

You didn't specifically request advanced technology to be in your life. It was handed to you whether you liked it or not. It was all around you as you moved from boy to teen to manhood, always advancing at an unstoppable pace, affecting your life completely. We can't turn back time, and living a non-digital life when you have responsibilities and ambition is quite tricky to do. But we can move forward with an important question:

- How do we address the negative side effects of technology?

In this chapter, I'll be unpacking four of the key issues around technology – pornography, the manosphere, gambling and social media envy – to look at how they impact us as men and why they are so damaging. And I'll consider how to create better digital habits that safeguard our wellbeing but without cutting us off. You might wonder why I've not mentioned gaming in this mix, and I've certainly met plenty of gaming widows (as well as golfing widows). I do appreciate that online gaming addiction is a growing people issue. It certainly affects more males than females, pulling them into hours of highly immersive and limitless play where they can be the hero, the tough guy and live out a fantasy life. But the research on the impact of gaming on men is nuanced, less clear cut, and it would appear that when it becomes a problem behaviour, it's more likely to negatively affect younger adults and teens, and this book is aimed at adult men.

Online pornography

In my teens, whenever I walked into WHSmith or any other newsagent, my eye would be drawn to the top rack of the magazine shelf, and a quick scan would follow: *Penthouse*, *Mayfair*, *Readers' Wives*, *Playboy*. I was a good kid and the son of a vicar, but I was also a teenager and, as a male teen, I now had 25 to 30 times more testosterone in my system than equivalent-age girls and was extremely curious about a whole new world I'd previously been unaware of.

If there were just a few people in WHSmith, I could quickly grab a mag and purchase it without dying of embarrassment. But the rational voices in my head would remind me that discreetly buying a pornographic magazine required a level of risk that was unthinkable. I refer to this today as the 'acquisition deterrent', in that the embarrassment factor of acquiring a porn mag was its own preventative measure – and it was highly effective.

As for videos, you had to go to sex shops to purchase them. There weren't many such shops about and I certainly didn't know of any. In WHSmith, there were two clear scenarios if I grabbed a mag.

- Scenario A: I would be refused at the till as I tried to buy it. Being refused the purchase and told to put the magazine back would be as humiliating as wetting myself in public while wearing beige-coloured chinos.
- Scenario B: Given that my dad was the Baptist minister of a large local church, someone from the church would probably be in WHSmith (because the congregation was literally everywhere at all times, and they'd pop up when you least expected it) and just as my hand grabbed the magazine, a church member would no doubt tap me on the shoulder.

I'd thought these two scenarios through many times, and they both made me shudder. The top-shelf scan always led to a wistful walk away to the birthday card section or the CDs.

The acquisition deterrent: it protected many male teenagers from the world of porn, and while we may have dreamed of a reliable, discreet and infinite supply of porn at that time in our lives, the acquisition deterrent was a complete blessing.

- There was nothing to warp my thinking and turn healthy desires into total depravity.
- There was nothing to create an addiction that would ruin any future sex life and mess with my head psychologically (and I don't use the word 'ruin' lightly).

- There was nothing to replace my brain's creative imagination, making it lazily reliant on porn and filling my head with unrealistic sexual expectations.

The modern world of pornography has been transformed by technology. You can easily find whatever you want, and it's in infinite supply. It's easy to hide your habit, erase it every day and start afresh the next (so you can kid yourself that you don't have a porn problem). With today's porn, you can even interact with the performers on sites like OnlyFans and pay to get them to act out whatever you want them to do. Today's porn is beyond an addiction where, at some points of the day at least, you could be out of reach: it's now all-consumingly available wherever you are. And what's more, if you're a male and online, even if you don't go out looking for porn, it will probably find you anyway!

The largest global porn platform is Pornhub. It's one of many porn platforms and its number of annual hits is hard to pin down, with estimates ranging between a jaw-dropping 60–120 billion hits each year (Merlio 2025). There are only eight billion people on the planet! And of course, porn affects both men and women, but it affects far more men, with 25 per cent of men under the age of 30 reportedly watching porn every day or most days, in comparison with only 2 per cent of women of similar age group (Kirk 2022).

It's fair to conclude, therefore, that most visits to Pornhub each year are driven by approximately four billion males. Bear in mind, too, that there are many other online 'adult entertainment' sites that also report billions of visits each year, and these viewing figures do not include the porn being consumed via WhatsApp and X. It's clear that those men watching porn every day or most days, really are watching huge amounts of porn: they must be, in order to generate such staggering numbers.

From young to old, pornography is easily accessible

to anyone with technology. In the UK, recent government legislation has forced porn platforms to apply stringent age verification checks, something which appears to have reduced the amount of UK traffic to global porn sites, but it's clear that at the time of writing this, there are still ways around the checks for those who are tech savvy – and plenty of men and boys are tech savvy, using virtual private networks to disguise their identity and bypass geographical restrictions.

Worryingly, it appears to be violent or rough porn that is the most popular genre. Analysis from the past decade suggests that 88 per cent of the most-viewed porn content contained acts of physical violence, with women generally the targets, and where performers expressed pleasure in response to the abuse 96 per cent of the time (Centre for Social Justice 2025). Add to this a report by the Children's Commissioner for England, that prior to the recent clampdown on verification checks, the average age when children first saw pornography was 13, with 10 per cent of children being exposed to pornography for the first time at the age of nine (Children's Commissioner for England 2023).

To put this into perspective, the earliest that I even became aware of porn was well into secondary school, when a single magazine with photos of naked women was passed around classmates (as if it were gold dust). Within that porn mag (or 'dirty mag', as it was known) there was no abuse, no rape, no rough sex depicted. Nor was it a limitless resource with millions of pages and genres catered for. The issues of online porn for viewers today (and in particular male viewers) are threefold, and I'll explain each in turn:

1. sexual tastes becoming more extreme for addicts
2. erectile dysfunction and difficulties reaching climax
3. negative body image.

Sexual tastes become more extreme for addicts

You may start out watching pornography because you're curious, lonely, bored, isolated and in need of an easy thrill. Maybe it felt harmless at the time and watching couples having sex was initially arousing. But as the weeks pass, you become desensitised and crave something more. You search for more extreme content, and it's easy to find.

You become addicted to the dopamine hit of watching porn, so your time spent watching porn increases. It's no longer an extra hobby on the side, or a nice-to-have. You carve out the time for your habit and family or social life comes second. With this daily consumption, the desensitisation ramps up, so the search for even more extreme content continues. It's a gradual journey into what I call the 'funnel of depravity'. It's not that you are depraved, a misogynist or a pervert – you're just an ordinary man, but you've transitioned into viewing genres of porn that you would have branded as 'disgustingly horrific' only 12 to 18 months before. You don't enter the funnel of depravity at speed or with clear intention: you slipped into it slowly, without even noticing.

UK comedian and celebrity Marcus Brigstocke has talked frankly about his porn addiction, describing how it changed his sexual desires completely, so that what he was into sexually was altered by what he was seeing – a testimony that replicates the reflections of countless former porn addicts (Butt 2025).

In a 2025 survey by the British Association for Counselling and Psychotherapy (BACP), more than half of their accredited counsellors and therapists working with male clients on addiction issues reported 'out-of-control porn use' as the reason for why men were seeking support. Among a number of problems caused by porn addiction were relationship breakdown and erectile dysfunction, but also the pursuit of increasingly extreme content. (Vinter 2026).

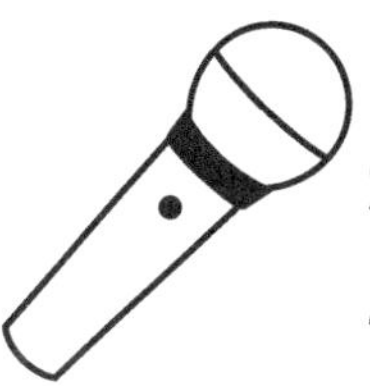

Shaun Flores, *Men on Show*, episode 48

> Shaun Flores is a mental health advocate and speaker, former model and former porn addict. In the podcast, we explored how porn affected his life. He said: 'The problem is, people forget if you watch the same things repeatedly, you build tolerance to that. You have to watch more extreme things to get the same dopamine hit and it continues to escalate. You need to go for more novel, extreme and taboo content to feel the same level of arousal, and that's exactly what happened to me.'

In the UK, there is now an Institute for Addressing Strangulation (created in October 2022). Call me a prude, but for me, the very fact that there is a need for this institute reflects a sad state of affairs. However, with 35 per cent of men between the ages of 16 and 34 saying they'd experienced strangulation during sex and 36 per cent of women in that age group reporting the same (Smailes & McGowan 2024), it's pretty clear that increasing levels of rough sex is a new issue. Proving cause and effect is complicated, but it seems obvious that increased consumption of extreme porn, leading to extreme tastes, is a likely contributory factor.

Erectile dysfunction and difficulties reaching climax

It's quite simple: the more porn you watch as a guy, the more likely it is that regardless of your physical health, testosterone levels or age, you will experience erectile dysfunction

(ED), and/or won't be able to climax when you are sexually active. It's another serious side effect from porn addiction, which was highlighted by the BACP survey I referenced. You'll experience no such problems while watching porn. Frustratingly for you, your body will respond perfectly to your PC, phone or whichever screen you use, but when having sex for real, your ability to function will deteriorate until you can't function at all.

A 2021 article in *Psychology Today* quoted research indicating that one quarter of men in their sexual prime experience ED if they're regular porn users (Weiss 2021), but before the age of internet porn, ED was mostly unheard of in young men. While most research on the topic relies on self-diagnosis and may be prone to bias, this same sentiment is repeated and shared in countless men's forums and porn addict support groups.

Lightbulb moment: Breaking the porn link

If erectile dysfunction (ED) is an issue for you, if it's getting you down (excuse the pun) and you're a regular porn consumer, I have three words of advice: ditch the porn! You could ignore my advice and try other things to sort your ED: maybe you get fitter, lose weight, drink less alcohol, invest in Viagra, but ultimately, nothing will work until you eradicate online porn from your life, and I don't mean 'reduce', I mean 'eradicate'. As a porn addict, your brain has become lazy and overstimulated by watching porn, so you'll need to go cold turkey and give your brain time to reset, which is months not weeks, but it will eventually reset (as long you don't fall off the wagon!).

If you struggle with porn, you are not alone. You are not a failure. But you do need to get rid of your porn habit, and for anyone who is still sceptical of how serious this issue is, bear in mind the study of nearly 6,000 respondents in the US, where a man's chances of getting divorced doubled if he started watching pornography (Shultz 2016). And, of course, as discussed in Chapter 1 (page 22), when we experience divorce as men, so our risk of suicide increases.

Negative body image

According to research cited in the 'Lost Boys' report (2025), negative body image is the most common negative effect on the viewer from frequently watching porn. Male actors, pumped with Viagra and implants to ensure they can produce lasting erections on demand, sporting perfectly honed physiques, fuelled by thousands of pounds' worth of performance-enhancing drugs: it's no wonder that so many of us consuming the content feel so inadequate. And if porn addiction is a growing problem, this is what we should expect to see in society today:

- rising levels of ED (across all male age groups)
- unsatisfactory sex lives and less sexual intimacy – because the sex is rubbish, as at least one of the couple (in a heterosexual relationship, it will probably be the male) are getting their sexual needs catered for online, and if the porn addict is male, his ability to function sexually offline will be getting worse
- rising levels of violent sex
- deteriorating gender division and increased gender resentment and mistrust
- increased loneliness (for men, women, people).

I'm gutted to say that from the media to my podcast guests and my work as a researcher and speaker, I'm seeing these trends now in society. It's already happening.

Tackling porn addiction

Remove the taboo from discussing porn

Online porn affects men of all ages, all professions, whether unemployed, successful, lonely or married. And yet, if I were to post something about porn and men on social media, I'd need to write the word p*rn (I can't even write the word, but according to the data I shared from 2023, nine-year-old children are accessing it), and I guarantee you that very few people would engage with the post. They'll be thinking: if I engage with a post on porn, others in my network will see my comment or 'like', and they may think I'm struggling with it myself.

As a society, and certainly in the UK, we generally don't like talking about porn. It's embarrassing, and that's part of the issue. The exploits of porn stars are reaching mainstream media for all to read. The story of Bonnie Blue's bedding of more than a thousand men in 24 hours was reported in 2025 in the *Daily Mail*, *The Mirror*, *The Sun* and *OK* magazine, and porn is being openly shared on social media platforms such as WhatsApp and Twitter/X. We need to talk openly about porn as men, understanding that if you're hooked, you're normal and not weird, but at the same time, it's not a harmless habit. We need safe, open spaces for men to be psychologically safe (more on that in Chapter 7) and dynamic communities of men (more on that in Chapter 8) so there is no shame in discussing online addiction, whatever the nature of the online addiction, and particularly if it's porn.

Quittr and X3Watch

If online porn is a particular issue for you, and you want to ditch it but just can't seem to sort it (and you don't want to ask for help within your network due to embarrassment), then there are a few options for accountability. You could try either Quittr or X3Watch (neither of which I have any affiliation with), both of which offer different levels of functionality, accountability and support to help you ditch the porn. As with all these things, the paid-for versions are much more effective. Do not make the mistake of thinking you can sort this yourself. Either reach out to trusted people in your network or invest in one of these support services: don't put it off. The issue will just fester if you do.

The manosphere

I became restless as a teenage boy. My testosterone levels soared and puberty began. I felt more edgy, cynical and inwardly aggressive. My musical tastes changed: Guns N' Roses, Iron Maiden and metal bands were in. Anything pop related was out.

My interests changed: bodybuilding was in (a weight-lifting belt with weights were bought and put to work). Cross-country running, which kept me skinny, was out.

My focus changed: girls were in; all-male groups like the Boys' Brigade were out.

Pretty normal stuff. But when I'd get home from school feeling angry about my unfair life (unfair because I was a late developer and very few girls of my age showed any romantic interest in me), there were no online influencers to manipulate that anger. I had no one to mislead me about how to fix these issues.

Instead, I had two older sisters who talked sense (and still do), and two loving parents with my best interests at heart (one of whom was always at home). We had one TV, one computer (but no internet because it wasn't available) and one landline phone. Personally, I had my Guns N' Roses cassettes and dumbbells to help me 'work out' my anger.

What I didn't have were voices preying on my immaturity and insecurities, capturing my attention, needing my engagement for their own profit, luring me in bit by bit, and taking up so much of my personal time and headspace that I might stop connecting with the healthy people in my life and be less likely to do the things that I really needed to do, such as activities to connect with other young people in a natural setting, or building my character and developing my skills.

Today, it's a tragedy that at a time when male puberty kicks into gear and our young men experience extraordinary changes in brain development (as well as a testosterone boost), we now have negative, misogynistic and highly influential social media influencers drawing our young men into their followers.

It's also a tragedy that as we become men and inevitably face setbacks through our lives – such as relationship breakdown, loneliness or financial strain, stuck in jobs we hate, feeling lost and inadequate – that these influencers are on our screens, 365 days a year. Because if the algorithms sense we might like what certain influencers have to say, then that's what our social media feeds will push to us, all day and every day: shaping our thoughts, fuelling anger and misleading us about who we should be.

The 'manosphere' refers to a network of masculine websites, blogs and online forums, each with a different emphasis. It's a nuanced space and it's not all bad: some of the manosphere is aspirational, motivating guys to take care of their physique or take up kung fu or boxing (and in my opinion, that's positive). But some parts of the manosphere are united in a belief that: a) men are victims of a society that is now designed for the benefit of women; b) that feminism has gone too far; c) as men, we should pull ourselves together and reclaim our power; or d) that we should completely disconnect from women.

Within the more negative side of the manosphere, there are also countless life-hack advisors and masculine influencers, peddling promises and solutions to dissatisfied men:

... The perfect body?
... Build a six-figure business in six months?
... Adoring, obedient girlfriend with pretty face and hot body?

If you want these things, just follow my plan and you can be the successful alpha male you've always longed to be. It's free today, but for the real life-changing stuff, and so long as you subscribe today, it will only cost you £28.50 per month! (instead of £329 per month).

The Liver King is a great example. He has a ripped physique, allegedly due to his 'ancestral' lifestyle, eating raw meat and offal, and he implored his followers to follow his ancestral tips (including eating raw bull's testicles). But he was later found out to have an £11k-per-month performance-enhancing drugs habit – the real secret ingredient for his physique (Weiss 2022). So, if you actually bought into his brand and followed his advice with gritted teeth, if you really did eat raw bull's testicles when what you really wanted was a straightforward pizza and chips, then let me say this: you've been played! You're not alone, but please learn from your mistakes. Just because he's online with a big following does not mean he has any credibility or integrity.

Then you have the Looksmaxxers, who advise you to maximise your physical appearance, either with soft-maxing measures, such as grooming, working out and mewing (tongue posture exercises claimed to enhance jaw definition – seriously, who has time for that?), or more extreme methods, such as cosmetic procedures, steroids or crash diets, or DIY enhancements performed at home. All of it pushed by influencers, most with limited credentials but desperate for a large, loyal online following, which might bring paying advertisers their way. Or the Men Going Their Own Way: communities of men online advocating for men to completely disengage from relationships with women and focus on their own self-interest instead.

More than 60 per cent of young men in the UK regularly engage with online masculinity influencers whose content is easy to digest and entertaining, and as time passes, it's easy to fall into the trap of seeing the influencer as a father figure and guru. If their advice to you is to take testosterone injections, steroids and diet pills, you'll probably do it, as others in your group will certainly be doing it and you want to fit in. As for the emotional impact of the messaging around masculinity, more than half of those engaging with masculinity influencers agreed that men should fix their own lives and not ask for help, and more than 80 per cent believe that men must be providers (Bancroft 2025). It's a form of messaging that simply takes us backwards, often when we're already struggling.

A word about Tate and the incels

Of all the individual influencers within the manosphere, Andrew Tate is the one name most of us have heard of, even if we don't know that much about the manosphere. A former kickboxing world champion, entrepreneur and social media personality, he has a massive online following, with more than 10 million followers on X alone. His content is a mix of champagne lifestyle, fast cars, physically beautiful women, six packs and biceps, self-help, autonomy and individualism, anti-establishment narrative and misogyny. Comparing women to dogs, he has previously asserted that women shouldn't be allowed to drive and that men have 'authority' over their female partners. He's also argued that women should 'bear some responsibility' for being raped (Will 2023).

From court battles, accusations of rape, organised crime and trafficking, to spreading toxic masculinity among our boys and young men, Andrew Tate's fame has seen him featured in mainstream media and even in debates at Parliament - which is why you've probably heard of him!

And while other Tate-inspired influencers have popped up to grab a share of the manosphere limelight (Sneako, Myron Gains, HS TikkyTokky, Justin Waller), Andrew Tate remains an influential figure at the time of writing.

As a 50-year-old, I can easily see that these influencers have little substance; they misquote history and politics to support their often-right-wing agendas, they spew misogynistic nonsense and promote dubious products and get-rich-quick schemes. But as a man, I'm at peace with myself; I'm privileged, happily married and connected in my community. For men who are isolated, who feel forgotten by society and increasingly angry about their predicament, I can see their appeal.

'Incels' is the other term most often associated with the manosphere. It hit the headlines due to the hugely successful Netflix series, *Adolescence*. But the series, while great TV, was misleading in its portrayal of the incel movement. The incels may share Andrew Tate's professed dislike of women, but there the similarities end. While Andrew Tate-inspired misogyny appears to be affecting young men, minors and children at school as young as ten years old (Adams 2025), the incel followers are predominantly men in the 18-34 age group (Whittaker 2024). They're part of a self-defeating, nihilistic movement that accepts they are undesirable and will never have a girlfriend or chance of being intimate with a woman. It's a bleak movement and highly misogynistic, but to young men who feel rejected, socially isolated, lost and cast aside by society, it provides a community of like-minded people, all of them suffering in anger and pain.

I'm glad the manosphere wasn't around when I was growing up. Now it's here and I am a proper grown-up, I'm glad I'm in a good place in my life: if I wasn't, it would be harder to ignore them.

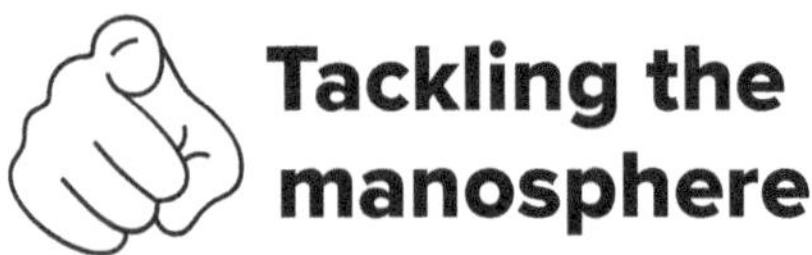

Tackling the manosphere

How would you know if your opinions had been manipulated?

It's not something that can easily be tracked. My top tip for protecting yourself is a long-term commitment to plugging into different *offline* communities of people. The more we become socially active offline, and the more we're cautious of just how much our views can be manipulated (however clever we may think we are), then we stand a fighting chance of staying on top of what we consume. If you're forming beliefs about something, don't take the word of one person (offline or online): learn to fact-check the things you dwell on.

Online gambling

Imagine that, just for a moment, you're transported out of the daily grind, away from boredom, from feeling inadequate and lost, and into a world of possibility: an exotic fantasy world that puts the spring in your step as you hope that, just maybe, your stars are aligned today. Josh Munns was my 33rd podcast guest, a podcaster himself and recovery support worker with lived experience of a gambling addiction. He described gambling as

> my escape place. If I had an argument with my partner, I would come storming downstairs and get straight on my phone. I'd go on a gambling site and would zone out. I could be on it from 9pm in the evening until 2am.

Once upon a time, Josh would have had to leave his house to gamble, either going to a casino or to the local betting shop. So, if he'd wanted to quit the habit, he'd have had a few ready-made obstacles to draw on.

Once upon a time, he'd have had to rifle through his pockets for cash, so he had a sense he was handing over hard-earned income.

Once upon a time, he stood a fighting chance of staying away from the danger zones (casinos and betting shops).

And today?

Like online porn, online gambling is available with just a swipe on your phone. It's there in your pocket and primed for action, which means there's no closing time or 'gone for lunch' signs on the door. So, if you're struggling with online gambling, rest assured, you're a normal bloke and victim of an age-old vice, which became a hundred times more addictive when it embraced the digital world.

I'd like to tell you that the global gambling industry is in decline, but the reality is that with an estimated annual worth at $540 billion, it's projected to reach a staggering $1.4 trillion by 2030 (*European Business Magazine* 2024). Yes, you read that correctly: global gambling is set to more than double in the next few years, and that growth is mostly being driven by men online. In a US study, 10 per cent of men between the ages of 18 and 30 were found to be at risk of 'problem gambling', as opposed to 3 per cent for the general population (Cassino 2024).

It's not that women don't fall victim to online gambling, but it affects more men, and the longer-term consequences are serious, with one in ten gamblers surveyed in the UK saying they'd previously contemplated suicide (Dugan & Crerar 2024). As well as suicide, problem gambling commonly leads to depression, substance abuse, domestic violence and bankruptcy (Moreira et al 2023), which is why the continued, meteoric rise of online gambling is not a problem to ignore. There is no shame in falling into this stuff. When life is bleak, it's easy to see the temporary allure and a small habit may quickly grow into something serious without the victim realising. The more we can talk about it openly, educate the next generation, and create communities where people can easily seek help, the better.

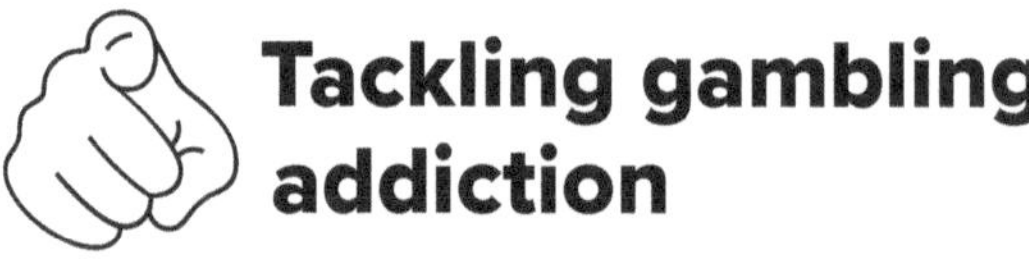

Tackling gambling addiction

> If online gambling is an issue, then you could try Gamban, which blocks access to online gambling sites across multiple devices, or Recoverme, which provides a structured recovery programme. You could try one or the other, or both. As with online porn, your access to online gambling is just too easy. Willpower will not be sufficient. Find an accountable partner and invest in technology that protects you from... technology!

Social media envy and comparison-itis

We all do it, yet none of us do it.

We *all* post our best bits to social media: the perfect holiday photos, out with the guys or ladies, big smiles on faces raising our glasses, the glorious sunset, quality time with Dad, the promotion, feeling *so* humble about my book becoming a bestseller (so humble, in fact, that I've decided to splash the news all over social media).

But *none* of us post our mundane bits (at home doing the ironing) and very few of us post our worst bits. I've yet to see a post on LinkedIn from someone apologising to their employer for the written warning they just received, admitting that the disciplinary measure was merited and that they promise to try harder in future.

We're surrounded by everyone else's best bits, exaggerated

bits and in some cases, fake bits, and there are serious consequences for our mental health:

- We feel dissatisfied. We were OK with our budget holiday to Butlins until we saw Uncle Steve's photos of his five-star, all-inclusive hotel in Barbados.
- We feel anxious. My university mates have already reached team leader roles with salaries to match, but I'm still in a dead-end job on minimum wage, with no hope of progress, living at home with Mum and Dad (when all my peers have moved out and have pads of their own).
- We feel impatient. He has a perfect figure, six pack, pecs, biceps and beautiful teeth. My own belly sags over my pants. I want what he has, and I want it by the end of this year at the latest. Where are my magic solutions?

And as for the time drain (which stops you taking action to remedy any of the above complaints), unfortunately for you, the algorithms know your weak spots. They know how to keep you hooked and coming back day after day, hour after hour. It's not that all social media is bad: there are positive influencers, groups affecting change and organising via social media, just as there are groups encouraging one another to commit suicide, do absurdly dangerous stunts for likes/followers or resort to extreme violence. But good, bad or indifferent, the screen time adds up, as does the relentless bombardment of messaging, promotion, information, oneupmanship and oversharing.

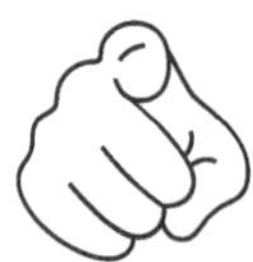

Tackling social media envy and comparison-itis

Maybe you don't struggle with an online addiction, but you check your phone far too many times, or in social situations where you could initiate a conversation, instead you grab your phone (in order to look busy and not alone: who wants to give off lonely vibes?). Now, I no longer reach for my phone. I have far more conversations than I used to have and these things helped me:

- **Switching off WiFi and mobile data as the norm**, so my wife or my kids' school can call me, but WhatsApp can't. I only turn them on in scheduled slots or if I genuinely need to (eg to book a taxi with Uber), but then I turn them off.
- **Phone in greyscale/sleep mode.** Each phone has the potential to be handled in these settings 24/7, and when you take the colour out of the phone, it's simply less appealing to look at.
- **One Sec:** it costs $9–10 for all your social media platforms, but if you're just addicted to one platform, you can download it for free. I used to be addicted to TikTok, but now, every time I try to log on, my phone goes blank, and One Sec asks me to take a deep breath and pause. It then reminds me of how many times I've been on TikTok in the previous 24 hours and asks again if I really want to open it up. To which my answer, more often than not, is no. (I have no affiliation or marketing deal with One Sec.)

Summing it up

Online porn, the manosphere, online gambling, social media, technology: these things aren't going anywhere. If you struggle with any of these issues, do seek help, do take action, do reach out – because your willpower alone is unlikely to be enough to conquer your online habits. Not because you're weak, but because so much of your day-to-day life revolves around online things, so switching off entirely from the digital world is increasingly less possible (unless you're thinking of living as a hermit).

6 The testosterone crisis

Sweat and rubber: these two components combine to make a smell I'll never forget, and when I smell it today, the memories of those places come flooding back. I'm not talking about a brothel (in case you wondered), I'm talking about a gym, but not a cardio-focused gym with neatly ordered rows of running and rowing machines. I mean a meat-building, sweat-sapping, cast-iron-clanking space, the rubber flooring absorbing the impact of dropped weights as shaking arms collapse. I was one of these guys, working out day after day, checking myself out in the mirror, watching the curves and lines on my arms slowly develop. You could almost sense the testosterone in the air.

If you'd asked me years ago what testosterone does for men, I would have said it makes men aggressive, risk orientated, predatory and muscly. I might even have thought that with less of it in the world, we'd get on much better together and the world would be a safer place. But be careful what you wish for. Testosterone levels in the male population are dropping, and in spite of testosterone's negative reputation, this decline really is bad news. There's far more to testosterone than aggression, sexual desire, risk-taking and bodybuilding. In fact, testosterone is so important for men's health that I'm going to make a bold prediction based on the research I've read.

Unless we can reverse the testosterone drop, men's mental and physical wellbeing will struggle to improve in the years to come, even if we address the other social and economic issues so far outlined in this book.

In this chapter, I'll start by looking at the evidence that supports the view that testosterone is decreasing in the male population. I'll then consider why the decline is such an issue for men, and then, crucially, what's fuelling the decline and the steps that you and I can take to reverse it.

Who says testosterone levels are dropping?

Testosterone declines gradually as we age, and because male life expectancy has increased in the last century, we should expect to see male testosterone levels falling to some extent (because there are far more older men on the planet today). But what's worrying is that testosterone is falling across the age groups. Let me just repeat that: testosterone is falling across the age groups.

I hate to break it to you men, but when your grandfather was your age today, and when his grandfather was also your age today, they would have had much higher testosterone levels than you currently do. The debate about exactly how much more testosterone they would have had is ongoing, but there's little doubt that male testosterone levels are falling. I'm 51 and it's not nice to think that my testosterone levels are not only in decline, but in comparison with previous generations, they are in super-decline. You may be wondering where the evidence is to support this concern, so let me stack it up for you.

1. In a study of 1,700 men from Boston in the US, data on testosterone levels was collected at three different

time intervals: a) 1987–1989, b) 1995–1997 and c) 2002–2004. For men aged 65 in 2002, testosterone levels were 15 per cent lower than for men of the same age in 1987 (Harding 2007).

2. In a study presented at the 2020 American Urological Association Virtual Experience, the levels of testosterone for a sample of more than 4,000 males between the ages of 15 and 30 had fallen by 20 per cent between 1999 and 2016. Even in males with a healthy BMI (body mass index), the reduction was noticeable (Kahl 2020).
3. A study of 5,000 Danish men found that the testosterone levels of those born in 1960 were 14 per cent lower than those of males born in the 1920s, with the number of men being prescribed supplementary testosterone rapidly increasing. If this is indicative of wider trends, then a general decline may have been in motion for nearly 100 years (Nordal 2020).
4. A study of 100,000 Israeli men between 2006 and 2019 found a 10 per cent decline in testosterone levels, a decline that could not simply be explained by rising levels of obesity or advancing age (Chodick et al 2020).
5. From tests carried out on Finnish men between the early 1970s through to 2002, similar patterns of declining testosterone levels were registered (Perheentupa et al 2013).

I could carry on with the data about declining testosterone – there's no shortage of it from around the world. Men's testosterone levels are dropping across all age groups: it's not fake news or a storm in a teacup and it's a global issue.

If testosterone levels in men are dropping, so what?

If, like me, you sucked at science as a kid, but you found yourself recently reading Carole Hooven's book *Testosterone: The story of the hormone that dominates and divides us* (2021), you may have found your brain aching as mine did. For non-medics, it's a challenging read, but a few things stood out (even with my artsy brain).

In the animal kingdom, testosterone fuels aggression in males. Outside mating season, when their testosterone levels are low, two stags can graze side by side and they're the best of buddies: it's a beautiful scene and the kids will love it. But as those same stags transition into mating season, their testosterone levels soar and they become mortal enemies who will fight to the death: it's like something out of a Quentin Tarantino movie and no longer suitable for the kids.

For humans, however, the impact of high or low testosterone is more complex, and Hooven makes clear that testosterone is not a magic potion that turns shrinking violets into angry warriors. The purpose of testosterone in humans is to coordinate male sexual anatomy (physiology and behaviour) for the purpose of reproduction. It's not a straightforward conclusion that high testosterone will create a risky, predatory and violent man, and beyond reproduction, testosterone is a hugely important indicator of mental and physical health for males.

- Low levels of testosterone in men have been found to increase the risk of developing coronary artery disease, metabolic syndrome (increased blood pressure, high blood sugar, excess body fat around the waist, abnormal cholesterol or triglyceride levels) and type 2 diabetes (Rezanezhad 2023).
- Low testosterone negatively impacts male sexuality, with

effects including low libido and erectile dysfunction, as well as decreased energy, depressed mood, irritability and decreased sense of wellbeing. In 27 randomised trials involving nearly 2,000 men, for example, testosterone treatment significantly reduced depressive symptoms (Walther et al 2019).

- Low testosterone is associated with chronic medical conditions such as dyslipidaemia (abnormal amounts of fats in the blood, such as cholesterol and triglycerides), high blood pressure, loss of kidney function and cancer, including the risk of prostate cancer (Goodale et al 2017, Xu et al 2018).

The implications of declining testosterone in men are serious and if levels are dropping, then we should expect to see increasing numbers of men dying prematurely from heart disease, increasing cases of prostate cancer and an increase of conditions linked to type 2 diabetes and obesity. We should expect to see rising numbers of men struggling with their mental health (despite the growing awareness about the need to talk and connect). And we should expect to see rising numbers of men reporting low libido and erectile dysfunction.

Sadly, we're seeing all these things right now and so, as men wanting to make the most of our own wellbeing while also looking out for our mates, sons, brothers, dads etc, we need to understand why levels are dropping and what we can do to reverse the decline.

Why are levels declining and how do we reverse it?

The reasons are varied, but modern life has created a perfect storm of conditions to drastically lower testosterone levels in men, including sugar and carbohydrate consumption, ultra-processed foods, with their lower levels of vital minerals and vitamins, lack of sleep and exercise, alcohol consumption, stress, low vitamin D, the plastics that are increasingly finding their way into our systems, and lack of opportunities for winning or otherwise feeling a sense of achievement. I'll take each of these one by one, first setting out the issues, and then some ways you can tackle them in your day-to-day habits.

Sugar and carbs

Do you find yourself raiding the kids' sweetie tin at the end of the day?

Do you need a mug of tea with a three-sugar pick-me-up in the morning?

Do you work night shifts as a nurse or on road maintenance, so a can of Red Bull or Lucozade feels like a life-saver when you need to get going?

Sugar: we can't get enough of it. Since Portuguese colonists in Brazil began producing it on an industrial level in the 1500s and shipping it back to Europe, we've got ourselves hooked, and for those of you fellas with a sweet tooth, I have bad news for you. The consumption of sugar trashes your testosterone levels. In fact, if you were to consume 75 grams of sugar right now (the equivalent of a standard-sized Mars bar and can of Coke), your testosterone levels would plummet by 25 per cent over the following 90 minutes (Diabetes.co.uk 2016).

You probably already know that to prevent type 2 diabetes and tooth decay, you should *stop* raiding the sweet tin, but you may not know about the link with testosterone. Why would you? Very few people do.

When you consider that higher testosterone will positively benefit your sex life, your overall muscle mass and heart health, are you sure you can't reduce the sugar you pour into your tea from three spoons to two, just for a month, then down to one spoon for the next month, and eventually to none in three months' time? When you analyse your daily food intake, remember that anything 'low fat' tends to be high in sugar, and it's amazing just how much sugar you find in 'healthy' cereal bars and orange juice, for example. And before you opt for sugar-free fizzy drinks, understand that these are not necessarily healthier alternatives and have been associated with obesity, type 2 diabetes, hypertension and cardiovascular disease (Diaz et al 2023). But it's not just refined sugar you need to watch out for. It's also about modern diets that are high in carbohydrates – and the remedy is to switch to a low-carb diet.

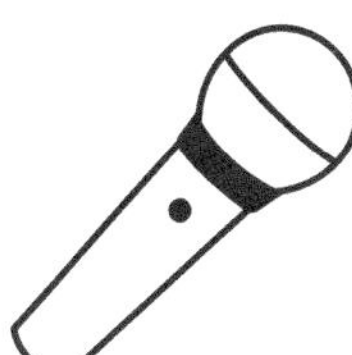

Ryan Parke, *Men on Show*, episodes 12 and 50

Ryan Parke is a men's coach, but he's not any ordinary coach. He's a TEDx and international award-winning public speaker, with an expertise in the science of men's health, and particularly testosterone. Working with countless men over the years, analysing their changing testosterone levels in relation to lifestyle changes, he's one of only two men to hold a seriously impressive accolade – being a guest on my podcast not just once, but for two full episodes!

In our latest podcast, I asked him: if there was just

one thing a man could do to naturally increase his testosterone, what would you recommend?

Ryan was unequivocal in his response: 'The amount of carbohydrate you eat on a daily basis is probably the single biggest factor. Carbohydrates raise our blood sugars, which contribute to insulin resistance, and this is probably the single biggest reason why most men now have low testosterone.'

In advocating for a low-carb diet, Ryan added that you replace your bog-standard carbs (such as bread, oats, pasta, rice, potatoes, breakfast cereal) with natural fats and vegetables: 'To avoid being hungry, you eat more natural fats like meat, avocados, fish – and also greenery so we get the vitamins and minerals our body needs.'

How to reduce your carbs

Rather than eating three slices of toast for breakfast or a giant bowl of cereal – both of which are great for convenience, but not so great as a low-carb diet – try things like poached egg and avocado, full fat yogurt with mixed nuts, an omelette or a vegetarian cooked breakfast. I'm a big fan of a poached egg with dry-fried prosciutto on top and grated cheese on top of that. If I have it with toast, it will be one slice of brown toast.

You could trial a carb-free meal each day or simply reduce your carb portions as a long-term commitment, rather than eliminate them entirely: two roast potatoes for your Sunday roast, rather than your usual seven; more sauce and less pasta (or no pasta) when you have spaghetti bolognaise; one slice of toast with your cheesy beans rather than the three you'd usually have. There is a simple two-stage equation to consider:

- Stage 1: Lower your sugar intake + lower your carb intake = rising testosterone levels due to lifestyle changes rather than medication.

- Stage 2: Rising testosterone = better heart health, better mental health, reduced risk of various cancers, better libido.

It may feel tough at first, but I'd gladly swap toast and sugary tea for those things. Last, if you're like me and you're looking to cheat only because bread is your best friend and cutting down on it feels like a step too far, then switching to brown or wholegrain is better than caning the white stuff. Because it's higher in fibre, wholegrain bread doesn't spike your blood sugars as significantly and will fill you up more. But be aware: you're still consuming carbs, whether it's brown or white carbs. Ideally you need to eat less carbs, whether they're brown or white.

Ultra-processed foods

From crunchy crisps in rustling packets to greasy double whopper burgers with buns that contain so many chemicals they could stay fresh for literally months, to baked treats, packet food, cereals: more than 55 per cent of the UK diet is made up of ultra-processed foods (UPF), with the figure rising to 65 per cent of children's diets (BBC Food 2019).

UPF food is ready made, convenient and nearly always cheaper than buying fresh ingredients, but UPFs contain an ingredients list as long as your arm, with weird and wonderful things that are hard to pronounce and you'd never stock in your own kitchen. The problem with assessing the impact of UPFs on testosterone levels is that there are so many chemicals in use within our food industry that analysing the impact of each individual ingredient on the testosterone levels of a decent-sized sample of males is unlikely to happen. What we can say with confidence, though, is that there are three food ingredients that are important for building testosterone, and these are seriously lacking within UPFs: vitamin B12, magnesium and zinc.

According to recent research (Panah et al 2024, Ciar et al 2011, Zečević 2025), your daily diet should be packed with these ingredients, and where do you find them? Not in a Big Mac, nor the packaged supermarket sandwich, nor the Victoria sponge cake you just bought, or the crisps and all the other things you love.

How to boost your vitamin B12, magnesium and zinc

Start moving towards a UPF zero-tolerance mentality. As inconvenient as it may feel, strip them out of your diet one by one and replace them with food items that are rich in vitamin B12, magnesium and zinc.

Magnesium can be found in the things you could have guessed: the leafy green vegetables, nuts and seeds, whole grains, dark chocolate (70+ per cent cocoa), fish, dairy produce, avocados, legumes, beans, fatty fish. You probably already know this and have read this list of food items in countless other 'healthy eating' articles, but if you want to reverse the testosterone decline, increasing the amount of magnesium in your diet is a start.

Zinc is in unprocessed red meat (steak, lamb, pork – but *not* sausages, ham or bacon), along with eggs, nuts, seeds, shellfish, dairy.

Vitamin B12 – think fish, dairy, unprocessed red meat, eggs and fortified non-dairy milk such as almond, soy and rice milk as options for vegans.

Sleep

This is one of my testosterone downfalls. Our boys just didn't sleep as infants: we tried everything and literally nothing worked. We're not alone. Even testosterone guru Ryan Parke described in the second podcast we did (episode 50) how his testosterone levels dropped when his son was born, with the only noticeable change in his lifestyle being a significant reduction in sleep.

There is wider research which supports the link between sleep and testosterone. When tested in a laboratory setting, the testosterone levels of male college undergraduates at the University of Chicago were compared based first on five hours of sleep each night, and then up to ten hours of sleep – and the results were clear. There was a 10–15 per cent reduction in testosterone levels when sleeping for only five hours (Leproult & Van Cauter 2011).

Outside the lab, US Army rangers from the 75th Ranger Regiment, an elite special operations unit, had their testosterone levels tested during military exercises. Now you might have thought that with all that exercise, dangers and bravado, their testosterone levels would be soaring by the end of it, but coping with sleep deprivation is a key component of the training, and by the end of the exercises, their testosterone levels had actually fallen by up to 25 per cent. Those rangers may have been fitter by the end of the exercises, but exhaustion caused by sleep deprivation negatively impacted their testosterone (Mantua et al 2020).

The sleep issue is a real problem for us blokes in the UK, because in 2023, a poll of 8,000 people found that the average adult in the UK gets less than six hours of sleep every night, with 10 per cent of those surveyed saying they get between two and four hours (Work in Mind 2023).

How dealing with your sleep can help

If you're worried about your libido, your concentration, your risk of a heart attack, it's clear: you can take action by prioritising your sleep, which will help you build testosterone. I appreciate that in some cases, knowing you're not getting enough sleep can feel stressful and thus make it more likely you'll be less able to sleep when you want to. Also, if you're a dad to young children and stuck in sleep-deprivation hell, I can only wish you the best: there are no magic, one-trick answers. It does get better... in the end. And if you're planning a family or your partner is pregnant, I cannot reiterate this enough: *sleep now while you can!* Sleep as much as possible, and when your bundle of joy/overwhelm arrives in the world, understand that babies were not built to sleep when adults do: a sleeping baby or not-sleeping baby has no bearing on whether it is a good baby or not!

Lightbulb moment: Tips for better sleep

> As a guideline, and if you're struggling with sleep, aim for seven hours each night, and come off all screens at least one hour before bed. Use an alarm clock rather than your phone to wake up, so your room can be phone free and, in addition, take it one step further by seeing your bedroom as a screen-free room. Laptops, TVs and iPads are banned! Prioritise your bedroom looking relaxed, homely and free of clutter. Avoid late-night snacking and daytime napping, using daylight hours to keep active, whether it's walking, chin-up bars, trips to the gym or gardening.

Sedentary behaviour and convenience culture

No need to open or close your garage door – it does so automatically. No need to grow your own vegetables or do any gardening – just cover it in concrete or astroturf, save yourself the hassle of mowing the lawn and buy a couple of pot plants to do your bit for biodiversity. No need to walk up six flights of stairs – there's a lift, stupid.

We've created convenience at previously unimaginable levels. Just about every action that once required some physical effort now has a solution that requires minimal or no physical effort. We've become sedentary. Both at home and at work, people are moving less, with a third of the global population now estimated to be moving below recommended levels – up from 23 per cent in 2000 (Strain et al 2024). The impact of an increasingly sedentary lifestyle, due to seated jobs, seated travelling and seated relaxation, is increased risk of heart disease, osteoporosis and obesity. Obesity plus a sedentary lifestyle is a big deal when we think about the testosterone crisis.

In a study of obese men, participants were divided into two groups: one group were tasked to lose weight through exercise and the other through reduced calorie consumption. By the end of the programme, while both groups had lost weight, those who'd undergone intense exercise regimes had significantly higher testosterone levels than those who'd focused on reduced calorie intake (Kumagai et al 2015). In another study of male adults between the ages of 18 and 27, men's testosterone levels were found to significantly increase after an intense 12-week programme of physical exercise (Devi et al 2014).

Ways you can build in more movement

Moving more is a challenge if your job requires you to be seated and is inflexible on working conditions; or if, due to living in a deprived area, there is less accessible green space or affordable activities; or if your neighbourhood is crime-ridden; or if, due to obesity, there are additional physical health issues with your knees or ankles. But moving more, increasing physical exercise and sitting less are key parts of getting fitter and naturally building testosterone.

I've tried to set myself rules through the day when I'm

working from home and sitting on my backside all day. I have a chin-up bar and every time I go to the kettle, I have to do a set of pull-ups or it's no coffee or tea. This ensures that I'll do seven or eight sets through the day on a chin-up-bar day. I also know that if I put the chin-up bar in place on the doorframe at the beginning of the day, I'm more likely to follow the rules and do the chin-ups, because the bar is already up there, staring at me as a constant reminder (rather than in the corner of the room where it's easier to ignore). And if I intend to go for a run but it feels like a chore, I know that if I put my trainers and shorts on when I get dressed, I'm more likely to get my lazy ass out for a run at some point, because I'm already dressed for it. I just need to focus on walking out the door (rather than going for a run), because once I'm out the door fully dressed for running, the likelihood of me then breaking into a slow jog to get started is close to 100 per cent.

I call this the 'shoehorn hack'. Complete an action step that's easy (such as already being dressed in running gear – that's not hard to achieve) so that the main action step that's harder (going for a run) becomes more likely. You just slip into doing it because you're ready for it.

Alcohol

Just as Big Macs, chocolate fudge cake and cookie dough ice cream will decimate your testosterone, unfortunately so will the booze. I appreciate it's tough and we might nostalgically look back to the 1970s, when the recommended 'safe' weekly alcohol limit in the UK was a jaw-dropping 53 units (how did anyone get anything done back then?) but the fact is, however much I love wine and beer (and I *really* do), my liver does not, and nor do my testosterone levels.

We've come a long way in our understanding of the impact of alcohol, and attitudes are changing. In the UK, the number of non-drinkers has marginally risen since 2000 while the number of regular drinkers has reduced: it seems that the message is getting through for many of us. But for heavy drinkers and particularly men, the data paints a bleaker picture. Do you remember the statistic from Chapter 1 on men's health and life expectancy? There are 2.6 million deaths each year, globally, from alcohol consumption, two million of whom are men (WHO 2024).

Heavy drinking is bad news for your cancer risk, liver failure and your testosterone levels. A systematic review in 2024 of 17 studies comparing hormone levels in drinkers versus non-drinkers found that while moderate to low alcohol consumption had minimal effect, heavy drinking was linked to significant reductions in testosterone levels (Moosazadeh et al 2024).

For anyone wondering why alcohol negatively impacts testosterone production, I'll explain in simple words with minimal jargon.

1. Alcohol messes with the function of the hypothalamus and pituitary gland and so reduces the release of hormones that signal to the testes to produce testosterone. (I'll try to remember that when I next fill up my wine glass.)
2. Alcohol damages the Leydig cells in the testes, which are responsible for testosterone synthesis (essentially a neat little system that converts cholesterol into testosterone).
3. Heavy drinking increases inflammation, which further messes up testosterone production.

Lightbulb moment: Ways you can approach reducing alcohol consumption

There is some good news for those of us who really do enjoy a tipple. So far, moderate to low levels of alcohol consumption are not linked to testosterone reduction. So, where you can, moderate your consumption, move to drinking at weekends only. If alcohol is becoming an everyday crutch, where having a 'dry day' or two each week feels like an issue, please do address it and seek help. Asking for help is a sign of strength and most entrenched habits require more than just willpower to kick them out.

Don't struggle alone.

Stress

Stress and testosterone do not get on well and in spite of everything we have today, from modern medicine to convenience, gadgets and technology, global stress levels are as high as ever, if not higher. A third of people surveyed in America in 2022 reported that stress is overwhelming most days, and a quarter of those surveyed said that when they're stressed, they can't bring themselves to do anything at all. In the same report, people who exhibited extreme levels of stress were more likely to turn to alcohol and drugs as a means of relaxing, and experience issues with sleeping – all of which can contribute to low testosterone, that's before we even think about stress as a separate factor (American Psychological Association 2022).

According to a Mental Health UK report in 2025, a third

of adults experienced high or extreme levels of pressure or stress, 'always' or 'often'. The consequences are obvious: rising levels of antidepressants being prescribed, with eight million people in the UK taking antidepressants each year (Schraer 2023) – up by one million over a five-year period – comfort eating of UPFs and sugary treats, sleep deprivation and substance abuse, all of which are bad news for testosterone. But stress specifically? This is where it gets technical.

Let's imagine you're exhausted because you're working long hours, you're worried about your job stability, you have debts piling up and you are not sleeping well. You can't see an easy way forward because your job options are limited. In that scenario, you might be aware of your own anxiety – the tension in your chest, the dry mouth, the finger-picking habit and inability to sleep. But what you're not aware of is that your body produces more cortisol due to the stress and consistently high levels of cortisol damage those Leydig cells I mentioned, lowering the levels of testosterone that are produced. Think of it like this:

Persistent stress = consistent cortisol = damage to Leydig cells = lower testosterone.

The other issue is that men have an HPG (hypothalamic–pituitary–gonadal) axis, a complex system of glands and hormones that regulate testosterone. But ongoing stress messes with this system, which then affects the pituitary gland's ability to signal to the testes to produce testosterone (Rise Men's Health 2025).

Why it's worth looking at non-chemical stress relievers

If we're often 'stressed', our testosterone production will fall – it's as simple as that. It's why the art of meditation, mindfulness, breath work, conscious acceptance of things you can't change, continue to grow in popularity. These are not fluffy things which real men should avoid: they're testosterone safeguarders for men. I utilise my weekly happy anchors. These are moments in the week where I'm so absorbed in something I love, I don't think about anything else and can look forward to them, however bleak the rest of my life might seem. For me, it's football and beers on Friday evenings with my men's community and diving off the boards on a Thursday (which is exhilarating, scary and fun, all at the same time).

Do you have happy anchors in place that bring joy to your life, connect you with other people and don't spoil your finances or health? If not, what could you do on a weekly basis? (Monthly is not frequent enough; it needs to be something that comes around regularly.)

Vitamin D

I was once blonde and fair many years ago (alas, my golden locks are now grey) but as a fair child, I learned to avoid the sun. But the sun isn't all bad and partly due to my indoor lifestyle today, I was found to be 'chronically deficient' in vitamin D several years ago. I had no idea, although I was a bit fatigued at the time and generally feeling low. But I'm not alone. Vitamin D deficiency is a global issue that is getting worse due to a few key reasons:

- an increasingly indoor and sedentary lifestyle, from working at home, to screen-based recreation, to more time in the car, on the bus, in an Uber and less time on foot
- sunscreen, which prevents our skin from absorbing sunlight
- obesity, because people with a higher BMI tend to have lower levels of vitamin D in their bloodstream, because vitamin D is a fat-soluble vitamin, so it's stored within body fat and therefore larger amounts of body fat can

sequester larger amounts of vitamin D, leading to lower circulating levels in the bloodstream
- an ageing population (as we age, the skin's ability to produce vitamin D from sunlight declines).

One in six UK adults is vitamin D deficient, 20 per cent of UK children are vitamin D deficient and an estimated one billion people in the world are vitamin D deficient (Department of Health and Social Care 2022). From bone disorders such as rickets to osteoporosis and increased risk of fractures, to muscle pain and weakness, fatigue, depression, slower wound healing, cardiovascular disease and autoimmune diseases, diabetes and hypertension, a lack of vitamin D is clearly a serious problem.

As for testosterone, there's research from Denmark to Malaysia which indicates that vitamin D deficiency may also increase the risk of low testosterone (Monson et al 2023). I should add, when we talk about cause and effect, the studies around vitamin D and its impact on testosterone are indicative rather than affirmative and there is ongoing debate about the extent to which vitamin D influences testosterone levels, although from the research, it's pretty clear that there is a link.

What you can do about vitamin D levels

Of all the factors so far examined, this is the most straightforward to remedy. While you can eat foods that are rich in vitamin D, such as mushrooms, fatty fish, egg yolks, unprocessed red meats, cheese and dark chocolate, we need more daylight and in winter and darker months, when it's in much shorter supply, we may need supplements. I take vitamin D supplements through the year. They're not expensive. Do look at the small print on the bottle. It's usually a tablet each day that you take on a full rather than empty stomach to maximise its positive impact.

Plastic

It's filling the oceans, it's all over the planet and it appears to have a detrimental effect on testosterone.

A study in 2025 by New York University Grossman School of Medicine analysed global health data and found that phthalates, which are added to plastic to make it more flexible and are commonly found in food packaging, not only contribute to inflammation in the coronary arteries, they disrupt testosterone production (Walsh 2025). It's not the only study to make the link: in 2013, research found that males with significant exposure to phthalates and bisphenol A (BPA) in plastic packaging had significantly reduced testosterone (Scinicariello 2016), with other research dating back to 2005 evidencing the same links. We've known for a while, but most of us live in blissful ignorance, or we don't care, or we've given up avoiding plastic because it's literally everywhere.

How to reduce plastic and BPA exposure

It's easy to take the view that we're already screwed, that the damage is done and life without plastic is not an option, but understanding how important testosterone is for male wellbeing, we should start making small steps. Cutting out UPF food, enclosed in its plastic packaging, may therefore have additional benefits for your testosterone levels beyond the food itself. Less UPF food generally means less exposure to plastics.

Ensuring that when you reheat and store food, you opt for glass, use tin foil rather than clingfilm and reduce your use of plastic as much as possible is a good start, as is ditching plastic bottles and using a non-plastic refillable cup.

The impact of winning and why it's more than just a morale boost

Just before I started writing this book, work wasn't going well for me. I'd had a particularly quiet few months, culminating in a completely silent week. No bookings, no prospecting conversations, no emails back from the clients I'd been trying to contact for literally weeks, no one returning my calls or picking up the calls. And on this particular week, it really got to me: boredom, fear of the future, frustration, disappointment – these emotions conspired to put me in both a foul and apathetic mood.

But every Thursday evening, I have diving lessons off the boards at my local pool. It's a bit of fun and you can tell I'm not a serious diver as I don't yet wear Speedos. One of the dives I've struggled to crack is a backwards dive. Leaning into a backward fall takes some guts if you're not used it. I'd been trying (and failing) for a few months, with plenty of slapped heads and shoulders from dives gone wrong.

On this particular week, when everything seemed so bleak, I finally cracked the backward dive at my lesson and came home elated. That small and insignificant win in the diving pool was not insignificant at all. It boosted my morale and meant I went into Friday and then into the following week in a much better frame of mind. It helped me to stop feeling sorry for myself and start reaching out to people with renewed enthusiasm and belief. Winning and men: it's an important angle and there is a bit of science to back this up.

In 2018, 38 men in their twenties went head-to-head on rowing machines in Cambridge as part of an experiment. What they didn't know was that the competition was rigged, so that the 'winners' were randomly declared and had nothing to do with who actually won. Saliva samples taken before and after showed that those men who believed they'd won experienced an average testosterone increase of 4.92 per cent and those who thought they'd lost saw average testosterone decreases of 7.24 per cent – a difference of more than 12 per cent just based on the belief of whether you've won or not in a rowing competition (Martin 2018). While a sample of 38 men is smaller than ideal, similar small-scale experiments have drawn similar conclusions.

In 1994, saliva samples of Italian and Brazilian male football fans were taken prior to the World Cup final (Brazil v Italy) and also after the game – a match that Brazil finally won on penalties. Among the Brazilian fans, testosterone levels had increased by a whopping 27 per cent, but for the Italian fans, whose team lost, it had dropped by an equally whopping 26 per cent (Susman 1995).

Loneliness, unemployment, the difficulty of achieving key milestones such as housing and providing for a family, the impact of austerity on people and communities, searing poverty mixed with rampant inequality, negative messaging about men in the media: I think it's fair to conclude that there is an extremely large group of men today for whom a regular sense of 'winning' in day-to-day life is not their reality. Given the small-scale experiments on the link between testosterone and winning or losing, perhaps it's not surprising that male testosterone is largely in decline.

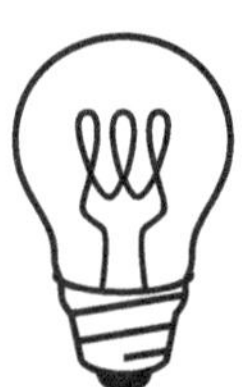

Lightbulb moment: How to win more

> **Set yourself mini goals that you can definitely achieve and call them out when you achieve them! I'm all for big, daring goals, and I'm all for achievable, daily goals as stepping stones towards the bigger ones. Share them with your buddies or colleagues. Create your**

own accountability group where you can share daily progress on achieving your goals. You may kid yourself that no one else would want to do this, but there are literally loads of men's groups springing up across the UK where daily sharing of mini goals is at the heart of what they do. The accountability will make it more likely you'll do what you promise you will each day, and the feeling of accomplishment will make you feel better and raise your testosterone levels.

Taking steps on testosterone

It's pretty clear that if we want to be in good physical and mental condition as men, testosterone is a key factor.

If you are concerned about your testosterone levels, the first thing I'd suggest is to get yourself tested. You can buy self-testing kits online from retailers such as Superdrug. These cost around £55 (at the time of writing) and if you have poor circulation in your fingers, extracting the quantity of blood you need for a reliable test is a challenge, as I found out for myself. But if you follow the instructions and post it promptly back to the laboratory, you'll receive a notification with your testosterone score (there are various factors which may skew the score, so you need to follow the instructions carefully). You could also get your GP to test you, but they may be reluctant to do so unless you're describing symptoms of low testosterone, and if you're tested and within the normal range, you may then struggle to pin them down to what your actual score is. Just in case you're wondering what an aspirational level of testosterone is to aim for, the answer is: it's complicated!

Testosterone levels decline as we age, so comparing the levels of a 25-year-old man with a 75-year-old man (or even a 45-year-old man) is pointless and it seems that age aside, there is no clear agreement on what is a high, healthy, low and dangerously low level of testosterone. That said, typical ranges start at 8 nmol/L and go up to 29 nmol/L. The British Society of Sexual Medicine recommends that testosterone replacement therapy should be offered to patients with levels below 12 nmol/L, with 18 nmol/L being considered a healthy level (Foster 2022).

In his book *How to Help Him: The book for women worried about a man* (2025), Ryan Parke details how most UK laboratories offering testosterone tests for men refer to testosterone levels of just 12 nmol/L and above as being ‘normal’, adding that with the NHS app, they draw the line of ‘healthy’ as 11.7 nmol/L and above. But here’s the problem. At the same time, Ryan also quotes research that indicates that for men with testosterone levels lower than 12 nmol/L, they are at increased risk of depression, suicide and prostate cancer. So how can 11.7 nmol/L be seen as healthy?

While testosterone hormone replacement therapy is a rapidly growing phenomenon, it’s possible to significantly increase your testosterone levels naturally, simply by taking action on the areas we’ve explored.

Lifestyle changes checklist:

- Ditch the sugar and UPFs in your diet, reduce your carbs and educate yourself on the real content of sugar in the things you eat. Low-fat products are often high in sugar!
- Sleep more: 7.5 hours minimum to 8–9 hours ideally.
- Move more: sports, hobbies, walking, activities at home: make sure you maximise your movement through the day. While we all love a labour-saving gadget, understand that there are downsides to our thirst for convenience.
- Moderate alcohol consumption: aim for weekends only and a consumption of weekly units that falls under the government guidance on 'safe consumption of units', which today is no longer 53 units as it was in the 1970s, but 14 units for an adult male!
- Find ways to manage the stress in your life, so that you're more equipped to deal with the bigger stress triggers and can reframe the more trivial triggers.
- Get your bloods checked for vitamin D and, if necessary, take supplements during the winter months. Get outside more, and eat foods rich in vitamin D.
- Reduce your use of plastics, particularly relating to your food and drink consumption and storage.
- Develop interests throughout your life that enable you to experience mini wins, so you're not simply reliant on work and money to define how successful you feel.

Part 2

How do we solve the issues?

7 Men and psychological safety

> "If you're operating from survival, you lose your creativity, and if you're operating from fear, it doesn't matter how good you are, you'll lose your ability to solve problems."

Harun Rabbani, serial entrepreneur, international speaker and mentor – episode 47, Men on Show

What do the words 'psychological safety' mean to you?

When I'm speaking at events and I ask this question, unless there are people from the wellbeing or equality, diversity and inclusion (EDI) department, it's rare that anyone knows. The two most common guesses people make are:

1. It's about people operating within their comfort zones.
2. It means feeling at peace with your life.

Neither of these are correct. Psychological safety is a relatively new term and it's a people game-changer. Other buzzwords will come and go, but psychological safety is a keeper. In fact, it's so massively important for men that I'm making a bold prediction: if we can create psychologically safe communities, we will have taken a huge step forward in safeguarding men's wellbeing.

Part 1 of this book explored the historic reasons behind why you and the men in your life might be struggling. I considered how the world has changed and whether stereotypes have kept up with those changes. I unpacked the reality of negative media messaging, the empathy gap, the need to celebrate male heroes and political laziness. I examined the various faces of technology and how it impacts us today, and finally, I concluded Part 1 by unravelling the complexities of the testosterone crisis.

Now in Part 2, I will focus on the potential solutions, looking at ideas and examples that I believe can help to bring real change – and the people who are making that change happen. There are four *massive* topics to unpack, and each is key to creating better outcomes for men. In the following chapters, I'll be sharing what I've discovered about the positive impact of men's communities, and how connecting with the next generation of men is crucial, whether that's through fatherhood or being a male role model. I'll conclude by considering how we think about masculinity and how we might update our approach so that it works *for* men, not against us.

First, though, back to psychological safety. I said that creating psychologically safe communities would represent a huge step forward in safeguarding men's wellbeing, and this is a bold statement indeed. So, let me unpack it by exploring four questions:

1. What is psychological safety?
2. Why is it important and who says so?
3. Why the specific link between psychological safety and men?
4. How do you create it?

What is psychological safety?

Rather than lift a boring, jargon-filled definition from a management journal, I'll share my interpretation of psychological safety, based on wider research and my lived experience.

Psychological safety describes the dynamic within a team or group of people where you feel safe to be transparently and respectfully yourself. For example:

- When you're psychologically safe, if you were talking about potentially sensitive issues with someone, you wouldn't feel as if you were treading on eggshells, because you wouldn't fear their reaction.
- If you had concerns about a project or a person, which no one else could see, you'd still raise your concerns even if you were the lone voice. You wouldn't worry that in response, you'd be belittled, patronised, penalised, ignored or sidelined by the wider group.
- If your relationship issues at home were impacting your work, you'd be OK to talk with trusted colleagues about it. You might not advertise your problems in the company newsletter, but you'd feel OK in reaching out to your immediate circle of colleagues/friends (or maybe a mental health first aider).
- If you made a mistake that you could get away with and no one would be likely to find out, you'd still tell people, because in a psychologically safe environment, admitting to mistakes, failure and weakness is normal. You'd know that by revealing your mistake, you might help someone else to avoid making that same mistake.
- If you had a great idea, but one that carried wider risks for the group, you'd feel comfortable to talk about your idea without embarrassment or fear. Even when presenting it to more senior colleagues, you'd be OK to

own the idea and shoulder the responsibility, because failure or setbacks in this context do not lead to finger-pointing and blame.

- If you had skeletons in your cupboard that you were ashamed of, you might actually take them out in an environment where you're psychologically safe.
- If you had a dumb question you wanted to ask that no one else was asking, you'd just ask it: why wouldn't you?

Psychological safety: it may sound idealistic, but there's nothing soft and fluffy about it, and creating it is easier said than done. The term was originally coined in the 1950s by the humanist psychologist Carl Rogers, but in 1999, it took on a new lease of life due to Dr Amy Edmonson. She published a landmark paper and was the first to create a validated tool to measure it, transforming psychological safety into the popular buzzword we have today. (Unsurprisingly her TED talk and book duly followed – fair enough!)

Why is psychological safety important? And who says so?

I'm a bit sceptical of new buzzwords. I agree that psychological safety sounds quite nice and that however tough we may think we are, most of us want to operate in an environment where we're not intimidated, silenced, ignored, humiliated or punished for our mistakes. But before we get ahead of ourselves in trying to create psychological safety, where's the evidence that having it in abundance makes a positive difference?

In 2012, Google launched Project Aristotle because they wanted to answer an important question: what makes our best teams so good? It's a simple question and one that people have been examining for centuries, but researchers at Google were intrigued that some of their superstar employees ultimately delivered underwhelming results, while other more average staff completely surpassed expectations. Google didn't mess about with this question. There was no box-ticking, Survey Monkey form or LinkedIn poll to generate impulsive and convenient conclusions. Researchers painstakingly studied 180 teams across the company, working with hundreds of variables (skills, personality traits, demographic, education and others) using more than 35 statistical models and a mountain of interviews. But they found no obvious formula for success: there seemed to be no specific qualifications, skills or demographic that gave people an edge over others.

Researchers then shifted their attention from measuring individual attributes to measuring how the teams behaved and communicated. There, they found five team dynamics that differentiated the best teams at Google, and of those five, psychological safety stood head and shoulders above the other four. Teams with psychological safety were able to acknowledge mistakes, experiment boldly and adapt quickly, outperforming technically capable teams who lacked such a dynamic (Schneider 2017). In summary, and according to Google, what may appear on the surface to be a fluffy concept is actually the beating heart of their most successful teams.

I arrived in London in the autumn of 1997, a fresh-faced graduate, full of hope and newly employed as a recruitment consultant. On my first day, I was still vague as to what a recruitment consultant did but figured that because my job title carried the word 'consultant', it would be a pretty cool job and I'd soon be making pots of money. From the very beginning, I had it drummed into me that experience, intelligence and work ethic underpinned an effective team. Success was about self-belief and graft, so work your arse off, arrive earlier than anyone else, have your lunch at your desk so you don't risk missing an important call, don't complain about anything and if life is tough for you, please talk only about your solutions, because we're not interested in hearing about the problems. People with problems need to get over themselves! Oh, and while you're at it, make sure everyone else sees your unswerving dedication and inevitable success. If the wider team sees that both things are linked, they'll be inspired by your example and they'll work their arses off too. It won't be long until the team is soaring like eagles: it's quite simple when you think about it.

Google's Project Aristotle challenges this assumption. Of course, the acceptance of long-term graft and sacrifice is important for pursuing long-term goals, but when we think about collective performance, it seems that other elements are needed to create success. Project Aristotle indicated that one of those elements was whether people feel psychologically safe and Google are not alone in their findings.

From corporate offices to the mountains – and I don't mean British mountains, which barely make the grade in height, but serious mountains, like the Himalayas. In his book *Rebel Ideas* (2019), Matthew Syed describes the research of Eric M Anicich, who gathered data from more than 30,000 Himalayan climbers from 56 nations and more than 5,000 expeditions. Anicich wanted to get to the heart of a key question. For mountaineering teams scaling the highest heights, does a dominant hierarchy increase the risk of disaster?

Just so we're clear on the words, 'dominant hierarchy' is essentially an absence of psychological safety, where if you're in the team, you shut up and do as you're told. You defer to a higher authority without question, and follow your orders to the letter. You don't bother leadership with trivial concerns because your leaders are far more experienced than you and whatever issues you 'think' you've spotted, they'll already have them accounted for and have in hand. So, accept your place in the pecking order and hold your shit together. From Anicich's research, the conclusion was unequivocally clear. Up in the Himalayas, where it's dangerous and uncertain, an absence of psychological safety substantially increases your risk of death.

From Google to extreme mountaineering, to the ordinary office life for that fresh-faced recruitment consultant working his arse off (but still quite vague about what he should be doing as a recruitment consultant), a lack of psychological safety negatively impacts your mental health, and I'll explain why.

The difference that psychological safety – or its absence – can make

I'll never forget Darren, who was my boss at that recruitment firm. He was uncompromising, full of management spiel and not interested in anyone's welfare (other than his own). However many calls you made yesterday, you can do more today and more tomorrow. If you were late due to a cancelled train, you should have foreseen it and taken the one before. It was an unspoken norm that committed people stayed late and got pissed in the pub together. It was a badge of honour. Every day, he'd wander about, pushing and goading for more sales. I'd see him heading in my direction and the pit of my stomach would wobble. I'd need to invent yet more excuses and fast.

My recruitment section was in trouble. No one within the organisation had worked that area before as a stand-alone section and even though I had precious little recruitment experience, even I could see that developing it was a long-term job, which is a problem when you have an uncompromising, no-nonsense boss wanting results today.

Darren's leadership style was old-school, macho male: a definite dominant hierarchy and not a morsel of psychological safety in place. We both lost out as a result, though, both Darren and me. He got excuse after excuse, matched with empty promises, and no credible insight as to the reality of the situation. The organisation lost out because the section bumbled along on the floor with no real prospect of improvement. And for me, because there was no 'we have your back' mentality or support in developing a patient, strategic plan to get things going, I stopped thinking creatively. I'd make phone call after phone call to the same old people, knowing it was futile, but honouring my call ratio targets set by Darren. It was soul destroying, ruined my professional confidence and at the same time, another issue started to bubble away outside of work: domestic abuse.

I referenced in Chapter 3 how I had a ready-made list of excuses for my colleagues to explain the cuts and bruises on my face. Within a macho, results-driven culture with an absence of psychological safety, there was no way I was going to say where those marks really came from. I was embarrassed that it was happening, and I was convinced that if people found out, it would put an extra mark on my back.

'Pain is struggling at home as well as work. He's a liability. Get rid!'

And if I got sacked, going home as an unemployed and fired recruitment consultant to my abusive partner (who liked to spend money) would have added to my growing list of problems. As much as I hated Darren, I really did need that job.

What if there had been psychological safety? How would things have panned out?

1. We would have explored the issues within my recruitment division and created a plan. I would have voiced my concerns about the time needed to develop it, felt supported and thought more clearly, more strategically. We could have carefully worked together, brainstorming stuff, experimenting new ways to get things moving. I wouldn't have spent hours cracking out pointless phone calls to the same old people who were sick and tired of hearing my voice!

2. Darren would have had an informed view of how to move forward with the section, rather than the weekly bullshit he got from me.
3. And if I'd seen Darren as a warm, approachable human being, who demonstrated his own struggles from time to time, I might have opened up about the abuse.

I eventually resigned and moved to another recruitment firm where the culture was much improved. Leadership was more thoughtful, but still there was no vulnerability. In the late 1990s and early 2000s, vulnerability in the workplace was unheard of and would have been seen as soft, and not in line with a successful sales organisation. As the domestic abuse continued to take its toll on me, so my work performance deteriorated. I saw the writing on the wall and hastily resigned. They were literally about to fire me. I beat them to it by about ten minutes. From Google to extreme mountaineering, to recruitment companies you've never heard of, psychological safety is a people game-changer: there's nothing soft about it.

Why the specific link between psychological safety and men?

When you break down the core ingredients of psychological safety, you could be forgiven for thinking it's just common-sense guidelines for being a nice human, something we've always known but which now has a label (and that label makes a few people a lot of money).

You could be forgiven for thinking that psychological safety belongs in management journals and organisational wellbeing strategies. Perhaps you think it's interesting enough, but you're wondering why it has its own chapter in a book about men?

There are three reasons:

1. Psychological safety vs the old-school man code

The ingredients that form psychological safety certainly help people to thrive – on that, the evidence is clear. But these ingredients don't mix well with traditional beliefs about how to be a proper man (beliefs such as: never reveal weakness, never back down, never admit to being wrong or not knowing the answer, never show fear). So, we may have uncovered a people game-changer, thanks in part to the work of Dr Amy Edmonson, but selling the concept to guys who hold traditional masculine views is not straightforward, because the essence of psychological safety clashes with old-school stereotypes. Maybe you had parents who saw good behaviour as obedience, keeping the noise down and not making a fuss, whereas bad behaviour was noise, anger, not sitting still when required, not listening or not following instructions. Maybe your parents focused on your academic and sporting achievements, nurturing a tough man who could make his mark in an unforgiving world, so discussion about how you felt and what you struggled with just wasn't an option. Maybe your parents weren't interested in hearing about your perception of unfairness, your feelings of inadequacy or fears of not fitting in because such conversations take time and lots of mental energy.

What follows from these normal parenting scenarios are stoical men, conditioned to bottle up their feelings and emotions first by parenting and then by a societal empathy gap that gets worse as he transitions from a child to teen to adult. Convincing such men that psychological safety is the way forward is going to require patience and solid evidence from compassionate evangelists. I'm a psychological safety evangelist. I invite you to become one too!

2. Testosterone

As you discovered in Chapter 6, testosterone is hugely important for men's physical and mental wellbeing. But there's something about testosterone that I didn't mention. It's not that I forgot to mention it; I just felt it was more relevant in this section. The Swiss neuroscientist and psychologist Chris Eisenegger has spent much of his career studying how hormones affect social behaviour, motivation and decision making. In 2011, he co-authored an influential review, 'The role of testosterone in social interaction', where he reframed testosterone as less of a 'violence hormone' and more of a 'status regulation hormone' (Eisenegger et al 2011). He has since revised elements of his work, but in general, his main points from 2011 have stood the test of time and continue to be accepted today. These points really matter if we want to understand why opening up for men can feel tough to do.

With significantly more testosterone in our systems than equivalent-age women, men are likely to have a heightened sensitivity to social threat, particularly threats that signal a potential loss of standing or respect. So, if we want men to avoid bottling things up, to go against years of parental and societal conditioning and talk comfortably about our struggles, then we must also recognise that on a biological level, it may feel harder and more unnatural for us to do that than for women – not because we're emotionally illiterate cavemen, but because of biology and, more specifically, testosterone.

Parenting, societal empathy gaps, testosterone: these things play a part, so if you find it difficult to express your emotions, because you either can't find the words or because it feels so alien, it's not actually your fault. You're not a sad, old-fashioned man in need of feminine modernisation. You're normal. You're an ordinary guy, doing his best to find his way in the modern world. It's because of these added challenges (parenting, societal empathy gaps, testosterone) that if we want men to speak up, to express their feelings and emotions, we must understand that for many men, it won't feel natural at all and will feel like lifting your head above the parapet, wondering when you'll get shot.

Eisenegger also found testosterone reduced general trust, because in certain social situations, misplaced trust could mean defeat or loss of position. The consequence is that men may be more guarded at first in social situations than women, and less likely to embrace an 'open book' or 'wearing your heart on your sleeve' approach in new social situations. They'll typically assess things carefully before revealing their innermost thoughts, and again, it's not because they're old-school men who need to get over themselves; it's in their make-up as men. There are exceptions to the rule of course and I fit the profile of an 'open book' type of guy, but research seems to indicate that talking openly about feelings and emotions is likely to be harder for more men than women, and that it's biologically driven as well as socially conditioned. It's why creating psychologically safe communities is so important if we want men to express their feelings and embrace the notion of vulnerability.

3. **Slow progress and the three-way tug of war**

Today, it can feel like, as a man, you're caught and pulled between three different viewpoints and demands:

A. Dear men, please open up about your struggles.
B. Dear men, if your struggles are caused by a woman, please shut up, accept you provoked her in the first place or if you must speak out, make sure you emphasise that you're in the absolute minority as a male victim.
C. Dear men, reject the modern equality nonsense. Feminism has gone too far. Reclaim your power. Your

trousers are there waiting for you. They always have been. Stop ignoring them and put them back on.

On the one hand, society has stepped in the right direction. In a recent Pew Research study of 10,000 Americans, nearly half of the men surveyed said they'd feel comfortable talking about their mental health with a therapist (Pasquini & Kikuchi 2024) and in the UK, the proportion of men attending therapy has risen from 18 per cent in 2010 to 29 per cent today (BACP 2025). Within our workplaces and communities, there is also a growing awareness that environments where people can speak openly and without fear will lead to better wellbeing and team performance. We really should celebrate the progress.

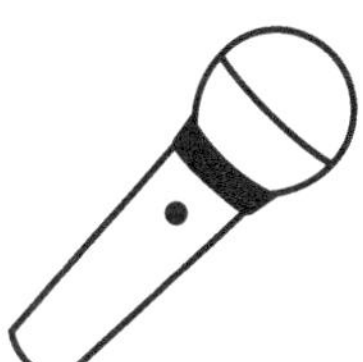

Stevie Ward, *Men on Show*, episode 25

Stevie Ward is the former captain of the Leeds Rhinos Rugby League team, part of their golden generation and one of the most successful teams in Super League history. He became the youngest Grand Final winner ever, eventually winning three Grand Finals, two Challenge Cups and named captain at just 26. When I asked Stevie about how mental health was perceived within elite Rugby League clubs, he was clear that at the start of his career, 'It wasn't really a thing. It was literally just relying on carrying out the physical task, without much thought for coaching and empathy and emotion. It's definitely sort of progressing and changing now.'

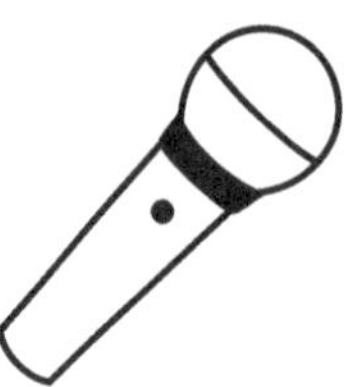

Ricky Nuttall, *Men on Show*, episode 30

> **Ricky Nuttall is a former firefighter and one of the first responders at the horrific Grenfell Tower tragedy. I showcased his story in Chapter 4. He described how early in his career within the fire service, they coped with the horrors of their job by masking it through dark humour, but how today, they're more likely to check in with each other in the cab on the way back to the station and be more real than they might have previously been.**

We now have more than half a million certified mental health first aiders in the UK today (Venture Zero 2023) and it's clear that overall, we're more accepting that everyone (including men) has mental health issues and it's variable from day to day. It feels as if we're finally moving away from seeing poor mental health as weird or weak and seeing it instead as a normal, human thing. But on the other hand, nearly half (47 per cent) of men in the Pew Research study I referenced still think there's a stigma about having counselling or psychotherapy, and a third of men surveyed in that same study think therapy is self-indulgent (compared to only 17 per cent of women). In a 2024 Movember report, *The Real Face of Men's Health*, more than 60 per cent of men surveyed said that traditional stereotypes, like 'good men tough it out', have affected their health behaviours and experiences in healthcare settings. So, what's going on? Are we moving forward as a society? Or aren't we?

It feels as if we men are caught in a three-way tug of war contest, with the first group of people imploring us to ditch the old man code and open up. Please *do* voice your feelings, please ask for help and *do* be more compassionate towards yourself. A second group is 'saying' the same things as the first group, but there is a crucial difference: if you're a bloke and struggling due to a female, then either shut up or be clear that this very rarely happens, or accept you probably provoked this woman in the first place.

The third group has an entirely different message. It's about recovering old masculine norms, something along the Trumpist sentiment of 'Make America Great Again'. Let's go back to the good old days, when men were men and women knew their place. It's quite simple. Toughen up once more. Get rid of liberal nonsense. Wear your trousers. Counselling and therapy are for pansies. Reclaim your dominance. Muscle up. Take no shit. You're a *man*, so embrace the old-school man code – you were better off in every department when you did.

This tug of war fuels gender resentment and creates confusion. As men, many of us already find the concept of being vulnerable quite tough to do (although we may be open to experimenting with it), but with the added uncertainty of how our feelings and thoughts might be received, opening up feels like too much of a risk to take. It's much safer to keep our heads down so we don't say the wrong thing.

Progress has been made in creating the conditions for psychologically safe spaces to exist, but until research can show that the vast majority of men could open up if they wanted to, and until research could also demonstrate that only a tiny handful of men would see counselling or therapeutic intervention as self-indulgent (ie 5 per cent rather than 33 per cent), then the job to create safe psychological spaces is a work in progress rather than mission accomplished.

How do you create psychological safety?

Psychological safety doesn't just happen. We're human, after all, and today's world is more complex, fast paced and uncertain than ever. We all have a public mask that sits over our private face (our real face) and taking that mask off generally feels uncomfortable whoever we are – and particularly for men, who may be less used to taking it off than women. But if psychological safety is as important as the evidence indicates, then create it we must.

1. Spread the message

When I'm delivering a keynote talk for your organisation, I'll be very grateful to you for the introduction you made on my behalf, but do make sure that you and your team know exactly what psychological safety is. After you read this book, part of your mission is to spread the word about psychological safety, and when you're reaching out to other guys who may still hold onto their out-of-date man codes, make sure you know a bit about the evidence. Old-school thinkers are likely to resist a concept that sounds soft and fluffy, but the evidence continues to mount up in support of its case for human wellbeing, excellence and innovation.

For a quick resource, you could check out Amy Edmonson's TED talk from 2014 on YouTube. It's only 12 minutes long, it's free and you could watch it with your team over lunch, then discuss what you think about it. Talk about it with your kids, your partner, your own parents, your bosses and peers. When you contribute towards the psychological safety revolution, you contribute towards creating a better world for all men (and the people who love them).

2. Give permission to be psychologically safe

How do you give permission to be psychologically safe if you're a construction manager on a building site, talking to your team of mostly men?

How would you give permission to your teenage son whose Xbox addiction and sloth-like attitude are driving you round the bend? Or your mates, with whom you've played cricket for years, but socially, you generally just talk rubbish and occasionally it would be nice to check in with how they're doing and get a meaningful answer?

There's no one-size-fits-all approach or magic solution, but there are tried and trusted techniques, which I recommend experimenting with.

Direct permission: Whether it's a one-to-one conversation or you're chatting with a group, you could say something like:

> 'Even if you know I'm in a terrible mood, and I've got a lot going on, if you've got something you want to share with me, something that you might be worried about (maybe you made a mistake? maybe you have an urgent holiday request? maybe you have concerns about someone in our team or one of my ideas?), please don't put it off. I want to hear from you, even when I'm in a bad mood. And if I'm grouchy in response, please say the words 'psychological safety', and that will be my instant calming down reminder!'

That's how I might give permission to a team of people I lead. Or maybe you're chatting over coffee with a mate and he says he's fine, although you suspect that's not quite true:

> 'I know you say you're fine, but you just don't seem yourself and you're my mate, so I care about you. Maybe it's nothing and I'm being oversensitive, but please know that I'm here for you: if there was an issue, please don't feel that it's so big or messy that you can't come to me. My door is open, I'm on the end of a phone, whether it's Christmas Day or my birthday.'

If you want people to feel psychologically safe, it requires the influencers and leaders within your team to take the lead and give people permission – not just as a one-off, but again and again and again. Make it part of your daily language, so it's drummed into your mates, your team at work, your kids, so people know 100 per cent that psychological safety is not a tick-box exercise.

Modelling gives permission: One bloke opens up; others sigh in relief. Because of that one moment of raw honesty, the other men are more likely to follow suit, realising that they don't need to keep it bottled up within this environment, and that they're not the only ones struggling to hold it together amid the daily grind.

- Maybe they're not the only ones who zoned out in the team meeting because they got bored and the spreadsheets made no sense.
- Maybe they're not the only ones stuck in a rut and unable to make their finances stretch in a cost-of-living crisis.
- Maybe they're not the only ones who tried as hard as they could and followed the rules laid out by online influencers, but nothing has worked: they're still single and in debt!

It's not that you have to take every opportunity to offload your problems on anyone who'll listen; it's about being willing to share concerns, accept mistakes, being OK with being wrong, owning it when you screw up, and understanding that this in itself is a sign of courage and strength. Modelling vulnerability sends a signal that if you open up in this environment, there is no loss of status here, because look, I'm already doing it and no one got hurt.

3. Manage your state

The problem in creating psychological safety for men is that they might be respectfully honest and the truth might hurt, or it might be inconvenient or challenge your narrative. It's not easy to be on the receiving end of respectful honesty, particularly if the other person voices an opinion that contradicts yours. And then there's the issue of time.

Have you ever asked someone if they're OK and you're *really* hoping they are, because if they're not, you don't have much time to hear about it – but now you asked and they've started opening up, so you're regretting you asked? This is the reality of psychological safety: shutting off our impatient 21st-century habits, creating space and time for people to be human and truly giving compassion and empathy the credit they deserve. A commitment to give time is at the heart of successful people and organisations.

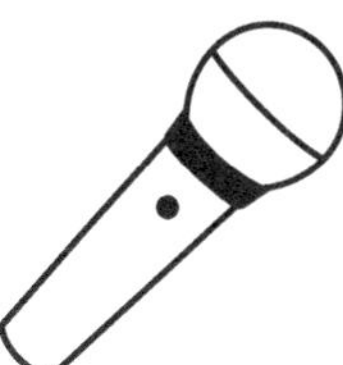

John Sidebotham, *Men on Show*, episode 38

John Sidebotham is a former wellbeing lead and EDI champion at Network Rail, and on the podcast, he discussed the impact on his mental health of being bullied in a former role by his female boss. When talking about psychological safety, he made this statement and it's a fitting way to end a chapter on why psychological safety is so important for men.

He said: 'The thing we can do to transform the world is to educate our children to be more compassionate. If we're able to practise more compassion in the workplace, it would be utterly transformational. When we bring empathy into the workplace and genuinely care for each other, we then talk about the bigger things that impact our wider lives and normalise conversations about our whole. Compassion creates an environment to thrive. It drives safety. It drives performance. It drives innovation, so why wouldn't you do it?'

8 Men's communities

It's a general rule of thumb that when you're a speaker at an event, it's best to avoid arguing with the delegates, because if it all kicks off, it makes it a bit *awkward* for everyone else. It's unlikely I'd ever be invited back, and 'word of mouth' can both bless and curse your business. So, as a speaker serving diverse organisations and often speaking about sensitive topics, finding the balance between diplomacy and authenticity is a fine art.

In 2024, I was delivering a talk for a men's network at a major UK educational establishment, and one of the delegates, a professor, started to angrily voice extreme views about women. My stomach started to churn. I knew I couldn't just leave such views without respectful challenge, but this could get messy quickly, like a runaway train with faulty brakes, travelling out of control. I steadied myself and was about to say something, but just before I could, several men within that network beat me to it. It was clear they already had a strong level of connection as men and a constructive debate ensued that eventually drew in quite a few of the guys who were in attendance. In the end, I didn't need to say anything at all. The debate was peacefully had, and I was able to move the conversation on, quite naturally.

But what if that network didn't exist?

What if that professor had nowhere constructive to air his views and nowhere to be challenged by people he trusts?

How might his views fester without such a network? And how might those festering views affect his behaviour towards his colleagues or students?

Men's communities: everyone wins from their existence; there are no losers. I'm not talking about a return to the old boys' networks of a bygone age with coded handshakes, closed groups of 'gents' leering over women and plumes of after-dinner cigar smoke. I'm talking about dynamic communities of men, standing shoulder to shoulder, supporting one another, holding each other to account and growing together. One of the most exciting developments in the men's wellbeing space over the past 15 to 20 years is the explosion of men's communities across the UK. I'm excited by what these groups offer, and I'm excited by what they can achieve for ordinary blokes like you and me. If we want to create better outcomes for ourselves, our mates, brothers, dads, sons, etc, the role of these communities cannot be underestimated.

You now know that as a guy, if you feel psychologically safe, you will find it much easier to talk about your feelings and emotions. You'll also know that as a guy, you have higher levels of testosterone than women, something that may make it more challenging for you to reveal vulnerability. You may not be used to talking openly and maybe you also work in an environment where you sense a lack of empathy for men. These things combined mean that even though you know you 'should' talk about your feelings, the doing of it can be really difficult.

Given that successive UK governments have been hesitant to make change happen for men, and at the time of writing this book, men's causes are hardly fundraising magnets in the charity sector, it's clear that men's communities have a huge role to play in creating better outcomes for men (and the people who love them).

I'm privileged to have interviewed some of the UK's best male community builders on my podcast, and this seems like a good place to showcase their stories and reflect on what we can learn. It may be that you feel lost, disconnected and need to reach out to a men's community. Or it may be that you want to do something for men but you're not sure where or how to get started. Either way, these case studies should give you some pointers!

Ben Mason: The Grieving Pint

Ben was the 23rd guest on my *Men on Show* podcast. Having grown up in a loving and stable family unit, Ben tragically lost his mum when he was 18. Ben had just started at university and his mental health took a battering from the grief. He tried traditional therapy but didn't find it to be a good fit for him. He didn't see himself as the kind of guy to sit in a counselling room with a box of tissues, but the things he really loves are sport and pubs (a man after my own heart, although he admitted to being a Spurs fan). Disillusioned with traditional therapy, he partnered with his fellow student, Alex Barham, and they created a peer space in pubs for male students to come for a pint and talk about their mental health. They started to pilot the space in April and May 2023, and the movement then spread to four cities in the south-west of the UK, eventually drawing in 60 volunteers (with more than 10 core organisers and 50 local leads).

It's such a simple idea. You or I could launch something similar if we really wanted to. A weekly chunk of time in the pub, where people who are struggling with their mental health can wander in for a chat, a pint, some banter and support or signposting should they want it. And if, as blokes, they've been conditioned to see counselling and therapy as something for freaks, losers or people in crisis, projects like The Grieving Pint offer an easier way to get started in talking about the stuff you're struggling with.

There's no cost, no NHS waiting list, no stigma, just blokes with open ears, ready to listen with a pint in hand. You needn't tell anyone you're going to therapy: you're just off to the pub! As with all initiatives, it takes time to spread, because it's one thing to dip your toe in the water to get started, but it's quite another to evolve it into a movement. But if you meet men where they are, if you tap into their interests, and you create spaces which feel natural and safe, then men do talk. It's an unhelpful myth that they don't.

Richard Loftus: Well Run Brum

Richard was my 41st *Men on Show* guest. He'd experienced a mental health crisis that brought him to a make-or-break decision about whether to continue with his life. Signed off work by his GP and prescribed antidepressants, Richard vegetated at home watching daytime TV, falling deeper into a rut, but then, without any previous passion for running, he got the urge to move and run. He put on his trainers, started running and never stopped (and by 'never stopped', I mean he is now a regular runner). His speed and distance rapidly improved in those early weeks and with a new focus, so did his mental health.

He asked his brother and friends if they wanted to join him and when he ran, he discovered something profound. It was easier to lower his guard and speak honestly while on the move, running side by side, than sitting directly across a table from a counsellor. Because when he was running, he was less likely to overthink what he was saying, and the words just tumbled out as he ran.

The positive benefits to Richard's physical and mental health from running inspired him to create Well Run Brum. Before launching the group, Richard trained through England Athletics, securing a 'Leadership in Running' qualification, to help him lead safely (and secure insurance), and then he secured a mental health champion qualification.

The first run took place in 2024 and Well Run Brum was born, hosting fortnightly 5K runs, drawing in between ten and 25 men. Each run starts with a guest speaker briefly sharing expertise and/or lived experiences on topics ranging from resilience to suicide and mental health crisis, then the men jog in Birmingham, and at a pace where meaningful conversation can occur.

Whether it's The Grieving Pint in a pub in Bristol, or jogging with Well Run Brum in Birmingham, two things seem clear:

1. As men, we want connection, we value friendship and we do talk.
2. We may find it easier to connect and talk openly in settings that feel natural. With both The Grieving Pint and Well Run Brum, neither has a waiting list or set of criteria to take part, which means anyone can join *today*, and for most people, neither group is financially prohibitive (other than the cost of a pint or a pair of trainers).

Scott Johnson: The Proper Blokes Club

Scott was my ninth guest on *Men on Show*. He'd always bottled things up when things got tough (as per the old-school man code), and he'd previously regarded poor mental health as a sign of weakness. But after a relationship breakdown, he was traumatised by his experiences of the family courts when trying to secure contact with his children and realised he needed help. He reached out to the NHS and was very positive about the support he was offered. He was first referred to a cognitive behavioural therapy programme, and while attending felt like a big step, after each of the eight sessions he felt much better.

Unfortunately, he was only permitted a maximum of eight sessions and then, in his words, he was thrown back into 'the wild'. He was at least referred to a local counsellor for additional support, but like Ben Mason from The Grieving Pint (and so many other blokes I speak to), Scott didn't feel a connection with the counsellor and knew that if he wanted to avoid medication, he'd need to do something different.

He started to walk for 15-20 minutes each day. The walking helped him to feel better, and so he started a Facebook page showing videos of him walking around his favourite local spots, talking about the issues he was struggling with. He wondered if other local men could resonate with how he was feeling. He hoped that by talking openly about his issues, it might help another guy in the same predicament.

After the first Covid-19 lockdown, he went one step further (excuse the walking pun) and put the word out on local Facebook groups to see if anyone would like to join him on his walks. The online response was massive, which led Scott to believe that hundreds of men would be there at the official launch walk, all of them ready to talk about their mental health.

On the day of his grand launch, no one arrived. It was a humiliating disaster, until at the very last minute, just one guy rocked up. They walked together, posted a photo of the two of them, kept going and the rest is history. The Proper Blokes Club is now a registered community interest company and has steadily grown to over 20+ walking groups across London, involving several hundred men each week: walking, talking and supporting one another.

Men's communities don't just happen. They need willing men to get things going and they need willing men to keep things going. Communities rarely just take off within a few weeks and generally they take time to find their personality, but given the ongoing growth with The Proper Blokes Club and so many other men's groups in the UK, it's clear that men value friendship and will talk so long as the conditions are right. And just in case you wondered, the 'right' conditions include feeling psychologically safe by doing an activity with other men who are also prepared to be vulnerable.

Christian Chalfont: Men's Retreats UK

Christian was my 27th guest on *Men on Show*. He's the founder of Men's Retreats UK, which very much does what it says on the tin. Christian's background is in counselling, a field where broadly speaking, no more than 20 per cent of counsellors/psychologists are male and less than 20 per cent of social workers are male (Secker & Williams 2024). As a male counsellor, he resolved to create a psychological space where men can talk openly without fear of judgement.

Set in beautiful countryside venues, groups of 12–20 men gather for the weekends, aided by fantastic food, no alcohol and activities including sharing circles, therapeutic workshops, breath work, cold-water therapy and somatic practice. On Saturday, they move into deep dives on personal struggles, and on Sunday, they focus on future goals and integration. Many of the men who attend describe feeling isolated in life, fearful of judgement and unsure how to articulate their struggles. They often report never having been in a space where men can be open and supportive. Common themes for why they're struggling include relationship breakdown, isolation, anxiety, depression and a sense of not belonging.

- ✦ What would happen if the communities you've read about so far didn't exist?
- ✦ What if there were no retreat opportunities for men seeking connection and support?
- ✦ How many men's lives might have been saved by the walking group (The Proper Blokes Club), or a weekly space in a pub (The Grieving Pint)? How many children still have a father but wouldn't do without these groups?

With an NHS stretched beyond capacity in the UK, add to that a lack of male therapists/social workers/psychologists, the empathy gap we explored in the first part of the book and the impact of testosterone, which makes it more likely men will see being vulnerable as a threat, then the existence and continued growth of these communities is critical. The very good news is that I could go on with example after example of men's communities, most of them thriving in the UK, drawing in men and saving lives. In fact, I'll do that. Let me introduce you to three more of my podcast guests.

Charlie Bethel: former CEO of Men's Sheds Association

Charlie Bethel was my 16th guest on *Men on Show*. I mentioned him in Chapter 4, referencing the issue they had in securing permission to create a shed in a space opposite a school. Men's Sheds is a movement that grew out of Australia back in the 1990s, its purpose to connect retired or unemployed men who might be feeling isolated and alone. The Men's Sheds movement is now a global phenomenon with more than 1,000 sheds in the UK, where men meet to fix things, make things and form a community (the movement is not exclusively male; some sheds attract females as core members). Amid the screwdrivers, workbenches and broken lawnmowers, men find friends, community, accountability and purpose.

Matt Hudson: Man v Fat

Matt Hudson, the marketing director of Man v Fat, was my 44th podcast guest. Man v Fat was founded by Andrew Shanahan. He'd attended a traditional slimming club but felt that the programmes were aimed at women. He wanted something that would really inspire him, and funnily enough, reflecting on menstrual cycles wasn't one of them. He started to think about a male-focused, football-driven weight loss programme that combined sport, community and accountability. Man v Fat was launched, with the focus on weight loss first, football second, and third, as a natural consequence of men coming together, community. Men engage with Man v Fat because they want friendship and a safe place to talk, as well as to lose weight, with wives and partners often referring men into the programme.

Man v Fat now has more than 150 football clubs in the UK, and the launch of a Man v Fat rugby league is under way. Thousands of men have lost significant weight, improved their fitness and built lasting social networks, and as for the names of the teams, they speak volumes about healthy male banter. My favourites include:

- UnAthletico Madrid
- Real Madras
- Expected Toulouse
- Rapid Viennetta
- Dynamo Kebab
- Man Titty

... to name just a few!

If I needed to lose weight and had the choice between traditional slimming clubs with talks about menstrual cycles or playing for Pork Vale in the Man v Fat league, I know which I'd rather do.

Patrick Nyarumbu: The Jabali Network

My very first podcast guest on *Men on Show*, Patrick Nyarumbu MBE, is the chair of the Jabali Network, an online network of senior male nurses with an African, Asian or Afro-Caribbean heritage. Nurses log in each month across the UK, their purpose being to create wellbeing support and role modelling. Starting with just nine men, they now have 100 members across the UK, breaking stereotypes, addressing under-representation both of men in a female-dominated environment and of men of colour in senior roles. Members report feeling 'psychologically safe' in a space where shared heritage and life experience mean that challenges are really understood. Patrick described an atmosphere of 'campfire conversations', where men sit together, sharing openly without fear of judgement and connecting on a deep level. That they have created such bonds through meeting online says a lot about their desire for connection. Of all the online communities I've ever worked with as a speaker, the Jabali Network is the one that stands out in terms of dynamism, humility and authenticity.

Across the UK, there are groups of men connecting with one another to form community, support each other and talk in safe spaces. Some of these communities are 'talk' focused, such as the Jabali Network and more widely in the UK, Andy's Man Club and Andy's ManGang. Others such as the Proper Blokes Club, Man v Fat, Men's Sheds and Well Run Brum are focused on an activity, where the aims are still connecting and talking openly, but while also doing something together such as woodwork, walking, running, playing football and losing weight.

The emergence and rapid expansion of these groups in recent years is testimony to the fact that men might be struggling, but they're trying to reach out and respond. The variety within these groups is essential. Men's Sheds would be no good for me because I hate woodwork and improving my diabolical skills in that area would require a level of time which at this stage in my life I simply don't have to spare.

I like to get outside, be active, play sport and drink beer, so my men's community is The Bearwood Dads. We live in Bearwood, we meet for a football match followed by beers each Friday evening and it's hugely important to my wellbeing. The WhatsApp group comes alive with banter on

Friday afternoons, and because the community is formed of mostly dads from my son's school, I bump into dads I know all the time. Aside from the weekly football, we meet for a meal every three months, and when there's a big football match on at the weekend, there's usually a few of the group out watching, and everyone's welcome. Sometimes we just talk about football, gossip and banter, but sometimes we talk about the stuff we struggle with. If you put me in a pub after a game of football, with trusted friends and a pint, I'll talk about anything and everything.

- Maybe you've tried counselling and it didn't do much for you?
- Maybe you wondered what was wrong with you, because counselling clearly works for other people, so why not you?
- Maybe you blamed the counsellor? Yourself? Or both?

Rest assured, there's nothing wrong with you. You're completely normal as a bloke, and aside from what I think, there is some research to back this up. There is a school of thought that follows the work of Deborah Tannen in her book *You Just Don't Understand* (1990), which proposes that women and men communicate differently, with women, on average, more likely to use communication for connection, expressing emotions and building relationships, whereas men are more likely to use communication for an exchange of information and/or problem solving. She describes it in her book as 'rapport talk' (women) vs 'report talk' (men).

Academics caution about treating her work as hard science, but if we can agree that as a trend, there may be small differences between how men and women may communicate, then Tannen's work might help to explain why the activity element within men's communities is so important in helping us to bond and talk more easily. Added to Tannen's work is the research from Eisenegger on testosterone, which

I referenced in Chapter 7. Eisenegger also found that testosterone fuels goal-orientated behaviour and reward seeking, so that men are more likely to cope and thrive through action-orientated strategies such as exercise and problem solving. If Eisenegger is right, it may explain why for some men, sitting in a counselling room exploring their feelings in depth just doesn't inspire them, and it may be something to bear in mind if you're thinking about starting your own men's community. It's also something to bear in mind if as a bloke, you've previously tried counselling and got nothing from it.

My Friday football has a primary purpose (football), but then in the pub after the game, talking about feelings happens – not always, but sometimes. The deeper stuff, if and when it happens, is a natural outworking of being part of a group who are open for friendship that extends beyond the game and beer. I don't say to my wife on a Friday evening, 'I'm off to therapy', but on reflection, maybe the football community is a form of therapy, but without the label. Whether it's running at Well Run Brum, walking at the Proper Blokes Club or socialising at The Grieving Pint, these activities act as social camouflage, which makes it easier to join in.

My tips for finding or creating your own men's community

Invite other men to share your interests

What interests do you currently have or do, which you could invite your mates along to? When you meet other guys, ask what their interests are and whether they want to join you in your stuff. Maybe you're a cook or baker and you're asking yourself: what guy would ask another guy over to his house to bake together? But maybe it's not such an odd invitation to extend: we have a men's pie club in the north-east of England with more than 300 members across 30+ groups. They've not been on my podcast yet, but they're active and baking a lot of pies.

I've been an active recruiter for my men's football group. Many of the men I invite don't like football, or they already play it, or they can't make it on a Friday, or they have knees that have had too much wear and tear. Occasionally, though, guys join, and I can think of two men I've recruited in the past few years, both of whom have both endured some tough personal times and seen the football community as a lifeline. Both are fathers. What if I'd never invited them?

Find a community (or two) if you don't have one

It's easy to lose contact with friends. It's easy to live a life where you've no one to turn to in a crisis. It's easy to reach a point where even for the fun stuff, you've no friends to share those moments with. Understand this: when we become lonely, our minds become our worst enemies. We get caught in self-inflicted lies that 'no one cares', 'we don't fit in' and 'people aren't interested in connecting with me'. These lies then make our predicament even worse. What are your interests? What do you like doing? What have you never done before, but maybe you'd like to give it a try? Whatever the answer is, *do it*! Reach out, take a small risk. You'll need to do the graft in the early stages because connection can take a bit of time to form. Get along to new things. Allow time for friendship to deepen. You may want a circle of friends *now*, but it takes time.

Form a community

You could plan it and do your homework first, as Richard Loftus did with Well Run Brum, or you could start small as Scott Johnson did with the Proper Blokes Club. Communities take time to form and evolve. Maybe your community will become a small intimate group: a group of four guys who didn't know each other before, but you asked around at work and on social media, to see if there are any mediocre and lonely golfers who haven't played for a while. You got just one response, but then a few months later, two more joined your golfing group and the group gelled well at four.

Maybe the initiative grows, and you initiate groups at different golf courses, with the focus on connection, mental health, talking and golf. You decide to call the group Men on Course. Or maybe the group doesn't grow. But even if you start something that connects just three or four guys, you may have just saved someone's life without even knowing it. In fact, you may have saved your own life without yet knowing it.

9 Men and fatherhood

I can't think of anything else as joyful, purposeful and overwhelmingly stressful (all at the same time) than being a dad. It might be that you're a stepdad, foster parent, or legal guardian, but if you've experienced the parenting rollercoaster in whatever format, you'll know it's an exhilarating yet gut-wrenching ride.

Maybe you're experiencing sleep deprivation torture and you wonder whether you'll ever feel human again?

Maybe your fragile newborn has slipped down the percentile chart for his body weight. He's now in the bottom 10 per cent. You're worried sick about the lack of weight gain, but in years to come, you'll be obsessing that he looks like Shrek (and fitting padlocks to the snack drawer).

Maybe your children won't stop bickering, except when they're on their damn phones and then they're completely unresponsive. Why can't they achieve a healthy middle ground? (It's bad parenting, right?)

As for the money that underpins all this jazz, it's tough for parents trying to provide in a cost-of-living crisis, particularly when society is so unequal. Add to the financial pressure the outdated notion that your worth as a man is still measured by the money you can earn, and it's easy to see why so many of us struggle. We could ask for help, but when we're feeling the heat, it's tempting instead to seek solace in bad habits that spike our dopamine today, but ruin our finances, health or relationships in the long term.

On the one hand, we want to be involved as dads and, comparatively speaking, we are. In fact, according to American research from 2016, dads with kids aged 18 and below spent triple the amount of time on parenting activities than their fathers did. In more recent research, 85 per cent of dads said that being a parent is either the most, or one of the most important aspects of who they are as a person (Cox 2025). We're modern men and most of us want to connect with our children. We want to support our partners emotionally and practically, and we know it's a privilege to have a career, especially when, for mums, it's clear that pregnancy still dents their career hopes. Juggling the pressure, the expectations, the guilt, delivering at work, yet being a dad and an attentive partner: it's no easy task.

In a book about men, to neglect the topic of fatherhood would be a glaring omission. It's a topic that has a huge impact on the current generation of men (fathers, stepfathers, grandfathers) and the next generation too (sons, stepsons, grandsons).

To do the topic justice, while keeping things concise, I'll explore three questions:

1. Why is fatherhood important (for children and fathers)?
2. What are the common challenges faced by 21st-century fathers?
3. How can we create an unbreakable connection with our children?

Each of these could form its own book, but I'll try to keep it all within one manageable chapter and take each question in turn.

Why is fatherhood important (for children and fathers)?

Sonia and Joel Shaljean are the driving force for Lads-Need-Dads, a brilliant and multi-award-winning programme based in Essex. Lads-Need-Dads mentors boys who don't have an active father in the household, and when I say the word 'mentor', I don't mean a maximum of ten 'interventions' then it's job done and on to the next boy; nor do I mean six counselling sessions within a six-month period, which nicely ticks a box. I mean year-after-year support. Working in collaboration with local schools in Essex, Lads-Need-Dads come alongside fatherless boys as they mature into men and they journey with those boys for as long as it takes. Sonia was the founder and now managing director, while Joel, her husband, is the education and training lead, and together, they're part of a team of 25 amazing people delivering the service.

Joel was my 17th podcast guest, and he described a pattern he'd noticed through the course of his work. At primary school, boys without an active father in their lives, he observed, typically feel sad and downbeat about not having an involved dad. At secondary school, those same boys now feel angry about it – something that creates disruptive, behavioural issues, the type of stuff that fuels the media headlines about toxic masculinity.

To explore this in more depth, the Lads-Need-Dads team collaborated on a research project, exploring the insights of 1,400 teachers, leaders and pastoral staff across a range of school settings. They wanted to analyse the impact of fatherlessness for boys, and the data makes for a sobering read (Hine et al 2022).

Primary school respondents:

- 89 per cent of those surveyed saw a link between boys with absent fathers (or limited access to a positive male role model) and disruptive behaviour at school.
- 68 per cent saw the same link with lower educational attainment.
- 47 per cent saw the same link with poor school attendance.

Secondary school respondents:

- 93 per cent of those surveyed saw a link between boys with absent fathers (or limited access to a positive male role model) with disruptive behaviour at school.
- 78 per cent saw the same link with lower educational attainment.
- 66 per cent saw the same link with poor school attendance.
- 60 per cent saw the same link with an increased risk of exclusion.

I'm guessing you're not surprised by the results. We've known for ages that fatherlessness negatively impacts boys in terms of their behaviour and school attainment. There is a mountain of research, but to add to the Lads-Need-Dads research project, a couple of quick snapshots include the literature review for the UK Government's Equalities Office in 2021, where it was found that a father's involvement in his children's lives improves children's emotional wellbeing, cognitive development and academic achievement. Plus research from the University of Leeds, describing a father's impact on his child's educational progress as 'unique' and 'important'. The research found that a father's involvement in his child's life reduced emotional and behavioural problems and helped to improve children's cognitive development (Weale 2023).

Not only is fatherlessness an issue for boys as they mature, but the impact also lingers on into manhood. Researchers found that depressive symptoms for men in the 20–25 age bracket massively spike if they have been fatherless as children and as young adults (Centre for Social Justice 2025). Bluntly speaking, newly qualified men first step out into the world with their future ahead of them, but if they've been fatherless as they've matured, it seems they hit rock bottom before they even get started. Could it be that in the defining moment of standing on their own two feet for the first time, fatherless men realise just how bereft they are?

The research I've shared on the impact of fatherlessness is a drop in the ocean. There is so much more I could share, but for reasons of brevity, let's consider another question. How much fatherlessness is there within modern society?

> An estimated 2.5 million children in the UK do not live with a father figure, representing a fifth of dependent children, and nearly half of the UK's children will experience parental separation by the age of 14 (Centre for Social Justice 2025).

Fatherlessness is a common phenomenon, with implications for the children as they mature into men. It's why the work of Lads-Need-Dads is so important. But what about dads themselves? What does fatherhood achieve for them? On this question, there is far less research, although there is some.

In a study of 881 low-income Black, Hispanic and White fathers, recruited from five states in the US, it was found that increased paternal involvement in the first year of the infant's life reduced the risk of post-natal depression (PND) for fathers – something that is experienced at similarly high levels as mothers (8–10 per cent of dads) but typically occurs at a later point after the infant's birth. Within the study, paternal involvement was defined in three separate categories:

1. Time spent with the baby or infant.
2. Parenting self-efficacy (self-confidence in being able to care for, make decisions and nurture the offspring).
3. Material provision.

When fathers scored strongly for each of the three above areas, their depressive symptoms were reduced. But when fathers were unable to spend much time with the infant (usually due to working long hours to provide), felt ill equipped to care for the infant or they were unable to provide, then the likelihood of experiencing depressive symptoms increased (Bamishigbin et al 2020). It seems that all three factors are important and yet within our working structures in the UK, often the third factor is contradictory to the first two. And as you'll have discovered in Chapter 2, following deindustrialisation and austerity, for many men, the third category (material provision) is increasingly difficult to deliver on.

Society has shifted, expectations have changed and it's clear that today at least, traditional stereotypes of a father's role (providing materially, working long hours to maximise income and leaving the parenting stuff to Mum) may not actually be in the best interests of the father or the child.

It makes sense when you factor in Mother Nature's intentions for parents, because nature appears to prepare men for a caregiving role as part of fatherhood. Within heterosexual relationships, when the female partner becomes pregnant and as the baby is born, so the male partner's testosterone levels decrease and his oxytocin levels rise (Saxbe et al 2017). This prepares the father for social bonding and caregiving. It's as if nature wants men to be involved in the caregiving of infants, rather than leaving the nurturing bit to Mum. So well before the dawning of modern civilisation, nature's concept design for parenting did not intend for new fathers to work 60-hour weeks, taking every overtime opportunity available, in order to provide for the family unit; and if there's one thing I've learned, Mother Nature knows best.

What are the common challenges faced by 21st-century fathers?

How long do you have? I could write novels about my fatherly challenges and some of the best and worst memories in my life are down to parenting. Definite lows include pacing at 2 am with a screaming baby who just won't shut up, night after night. Whatever we tried (Classic FM, soothing singing, pacing, sitting still, change of room, putting the baby down, picking him up), literally nothing worked. And yet the wider show must go on: housework, employment, parenting your other children (which for us included teenagers), shopping. None of this stops because you have a baby to look after. For each of my boys, it wasn't until the 15- to 18-month stage that things improved sleep-wise.

There is no manual that can prepare you for this stuff, and life does not return to normal when they start school. On the one day of the week when you and your partner (if you have one) both have crucial meetings to attend, that will definitely be the day that your six-year-old vomits all over the classroom. They'll then need to be picked up from school ASAP. Your employer 'understands' on one level but also makes clear that it's a definite blow that you can't attend the meeting. Plagued with guilt, you pick up your sickly kid and as soon as they're home, they feel fine, but school won't have them back for at least 48 hours and you can sense that your work colleagues are pissed off with you.

Even if the kids are rarely ill and you're a well-organised parent, someone has to get them to school by 08:40 and pick them up by 15:15. Breakfast clubs and after-school clubs aren't cheap, and they don't run much before 07:30 or after 17:30. The commitment is long term, the upheaval is long term and most of us are winging it as dads. We're finding our way, doing our best, yet feeling as if we're failing in our roles as lovers, partners, fathers and employees, while our body weight piles on because we ditched our hobbies due to time and finance.

But beyond the general chaos, there are four aspects of fatherhood that warrant special attention, because their impact is serious and under-recognised. These are:

1. Male post-natal depression (PND).
2. Physical and mental health issues for new fathers.
3. The family courts system (here talking about the UK specifically).
4. Paternity leave.

Dads and post-natal depression (PND)

As a father of five, I understand why post-natal depression (PND) is common for dads. And sadly, from years of speaking on men's wellbeing, it's no surprise also that it's not more widely recognised within the healthcare arena (we can thank political laziness and the empathy gap for that!).

For dads, there are the obvious challenges I just identified and then there's the less obvious stuff such as nature's changes to our male hormones following the birth of a baby, including testosterone, oestrogen, cortisol, vasopressin and prolactin (Kim & Swain 2007). There's also the subtle undercurrent of being ignored or sidelined as the father by healthcare professionals.

An article published by the Men and Boys Coalition (Miller 2025) described how the NHS website mentioned PND affecting mums and dads, but the information provided on the website caters for mothers and there is very little reference to dads. The coalition also raised concerns about the messaging from the National Institute for Health & Care Excellence (NICE). The NICE guidelines advise doctors to undertake postnatal checks on women's physical and psychological wellbeing up to six to eight weeks after giving birth, but there are no recommendations made for supporting fathers. Health visits are set for one to two weeks and six to eight weeks following the birth, but the research is clear that, for fathers at least, the most likely time he'll struggle with PND is from three to six months after the birth of the infant. But after the eight-week check, there are no further mandatory health visits until the nine- to 12-month mark. Even if healthcare visitors remembered to ask Dad how he's doing, unless PND is more widely recognised as a common condition for dads too, it's likely that Dad would just say he's fine because he's unaware that PND is a thing, so he'll just soldier on – no point in making a fuss.

If PND was vanishingly rare for dads, you could argue that for the sake of a few unlucky people, it's not worth the airtime. But in a meta-analysis involving more than one million participants across more than 30 countries, the rates of PND for fathers varied between 8 and 10 per cent (Alvarez-Garcia et al 2024). That's roughly one in ten dads across the globe suffering from PND, with knock-on effects for Mum and the infant. If we want to empower men to be effective fathers, then we need to be more aware about PND, so those men who are struggling know they're not alone or 'failing'.

Not only is PND more common than many of us realise, it's serious. Research cited in the *British Journal of Midwifery* (Hanley & Williams 2020) put new fathers with mental health challenges at 50 times more likely to pose a suicide risk than at any other time in their lives. Describing factors such as sleep deprivation, societal pressures, fatigue and witnessing a traumatic birth where, as the father, he felt powerless to help, the article recommended that fathers are included in policies and in the pathway of care to support all parents.

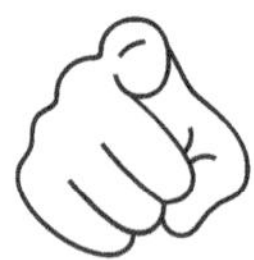

What we can do to tackle PND in fathers

- ✦ A good starting point for progress could include recommended checks for Dad's wellbeing as part of best practice (particularly at the three- to six-month period) as well as an updated NHS website, with clear information on why and when PND affects men.
- ✦ The UK government could improve the paternity leave offering (more on that shortly).
- ✦ As employers, we could ensure that our policies and procedures are fit for purpose within our wellbeing and parental leave offering. We could promote health and mental health checks on dads within the PND risk zone (at three to six months after the infant is born) and we can commit to making adjustments to prevent PND.
- ✦ Within our own circles, when our mate, son or brother becomes a proud father, make a note to see how he is doing at three months, four months, five months and six months. PND is too common to ignore. Empower a father, reduce the risk of PND and the ripple effect across his family unit will be profoundly positive. It's a step forward for everyone.

Dads 'letting themselves go'

Citing a poll of 5,000 men, the BBC reported that the average dad piles on a full stone of weight during his partner's pregnancy, due to making the most of their time together before the baby arrives (so more eating out, more trips to the pub), and an abundance of those pregnancy favourite snacks in the home. However, only a third of dads join their partners in post-pregnancy diets (BBC News 2009)!

It's a noble cause: mother and baby first (as per the Birkenhead drill), provision joint first with mother and baby (as per the man-code), and anything for Dad is firmly last (as per the empathy gap). Not all fathers subscribe to this model, of course, but as decent men transitioning into fathers and who want to step up to the plate, most of us wouldn't argue with it.

A more recent study from 2020–22 supports the findings of this much older BBC article, where new fathers were again found to be at higher risk of obesity and of adopting less healthy lifestyle behaviours (Whooten et al 2023). It's not rocket science. Scott Mair was my 36th guest on *Men on Show* and is the director of Fatherhood Solutions, delivering parent and infant mental health projects in the UK, collaborating with local authorities and maternity services. As a former military man, he described how as part of his job, he believed he had experienced sleep deprivation training... that was until he had kids!

I feel his pain. I feel your pain, too. I can only describe baby-induced sleep deprivation as a living hell, and not one that passes quickly. Of course, there is the joy and wonder of a newborn, but that joy comes at a huge cost to the parents, who are too tired to socialise, too tired to initiate new things, too tired to draw on the self-discipline you need to resist the sugary snacks, the crisps, the white buttered toast and glasses of wine by 4 pm. These feel like life-savers at this stage of your life. But time soon passes, your bad habits become the 'new you' and several areas of your life now drift. If this sounds familiar, ask yourself:

- As an absolute minimum, is there just one thing you could do for yourself regularly, something that won't ruin your health, finances or relationship with your partner, and something that would bring you great joy and completely absorb your focus when you do it?

For me it's weekly football. Through each of my boys' first year of life, that was the one thing I committed to each week (unless I was dashing to A&E). It was the one precious moment of the week when I temporarily forgot about nappies, the mountains of washing to deal with or the screaming babies at 3 am.

Do not underestimate the burden that fatherhood carries. Check in with your mates. You're not being nosy or a nag. You're being a mate. Encourage him to reconnect with old social circles/hobbies/sport. And if he seems reluctant, do not give up on him.

Dads and the family courts

When we talk about fatherhood, it's worth remembering that not all dads live with their kids, and of these not all of them still see their kids, and if they do, their access may rest on delicate ground.

More than 250,000 new cases come into the UK family courts each year, each case with its own complexity, pain and trauma (Ministry of Justice 2024). No one wins in the family courts. Decisions are often arbitrary and even when court orders are made at great financial and emotional cost to the parents, they're often not adhered to.

To avoid writing an unfathomably long section about the family courts, I'll make a few succinct points, based on my experiences from my own family court battles. You might be struggling as a dad within the system and I want you to know that you're not alone.

For transparency, in my first family court saga, my ex-partner blocked all means of contact with my daughters for three months until it was restored by the courts (by contact, I'm referring to the fortnightly weekends when they stayed with me, plus all phone calls, letters and emails. She really did block all means of contact). My ex had claimed that months before, when I took my daughters on a two-week family holiday abroad during the summer holidays, I'd actually kidnapped them. Whipped up by friends/followers on Twitter-as-it-was, she used the kidnap allegation as the basis for blocking my contact. It was an odd claim, given that we'd peacefully agreed the holiday dates together months before the holiday, she'd given me the girls' passports for the holiday, she had the details of where we were staying, the flight details for the outgoing and returning flights, and in fact welcomed our daughters home at the airport (with welcome-home banners and neighbours in tow). Not much of a kidnap, then!

We got stuck in the family courts for six months where, aside from restoring contact, I secured residency of both girls in the process. Both girls then moved to my care. In the second family court saga, four years later, my ex was trying to overturn this original decision and force the girls back into her care whether they liked it or not. She was also trying to have me fined and/or imprisoned for parental alienation, as both girls (teenagers at that point) were now refusing to see her. Both battles took up roughly three years of time collectively speaking and both cost me dearly, emotionally and financially.

If we're talking about fathers and wellbeing, the group of men whose voices are not often heard within that conversation are those who don't see their children. Bearing in mind the points made earlier in this chapter about a father's mental health and contact with his children, and the impact of fatherlessness on the next generation of men, we should be very concerned for the welfare of those who don't see their kids, or those who may still see them, but whose time with the kids is limited and resting on shaky ground.

The courts are a lottery: Whatever has led to your case entering the family courts, the outcome will be greatly shaped by the attitude of the judge and the Children and Family Court Advisory Service (CAFCASS) case workers. For the uninitiated, the role of CAFCASS is to understand the details and context of the case, so they can make independent recommendations to the judge, whose reading time on your case notes could be *very* limited (although finding data to evidence how long judges spend in reading time for cases is virtually impossible).

When I met with current CAFCASS CEO Jacky Tiotto, prior to speaking at the CAFCASS national conference in 2021, she referenced the more than 1,400 case workers they employ around the UK. In terms of personalities, biases, skills, calibre, old-school approach versus progressive approach, black-and-white world view versus balanced and grey world view, there will obviously be variance among the case workers who deliver the CAFCASS service. You may have a brilliantly insightful CAFCASS officer, or you may have someone from the dark ages who should probably have retired years ago.

The courts are unpredictable: Let's imagine that your half-hour hearing is scheduled for 09:30 and the court is only a stone's throw from your office, so you make the mistake of only requesting a half day of annual leave. In reality, the hearing will probably be delayed until 14:30 and you could be in there for two hours or five minutes. And when the CAFCASS case worker phones you during working hours, to help them consider their approach, that call might be 20 minutes or two hours and if they've already spoken to your ex, you're probably in for a very tough call. Your lawyer may also need a response from you on something important... *today*.

For all employers reading this, please bear in mind that the family courts are unpredictable and overwhelming. If you have a dad going through it on your team, he'll be trying to hold down a job to help pay for the court process (which ultimately could cost anything from £5,000 to £100,000).

Parental alienation and mediation: Parental alienation is the term used to describe one parent trying to spoil the relationship of the child(ren) with the other parent, either through badmouthing that parent or frustrating or blocking contact. Mums and dads do it. It's not a gender issue, but if you're trying to co-parent with an alienating, bitter ex, the courts won't have much sympathy. They will still expect you to mediate and negotiate reasonably, and if the behaviour of your ex is erratic and causing issues for the kids (and you), you will still be expected to *always* parent neutrally and without any slip-ups. The pressure, the stakes, the acrimony: it's overwhelming.

There is very little research about the impact of parental alienation on the risk of men dying by suicide, but according to a study in America from 2019 (Harman et al 2019), half of alienated parents surveyed had contemplated suicide.

What we can do for those going through the family courts: If you're going through the family courts or experiencing parental alienation, or know someone who is, then I have three suggestions:

- **Employers:** Do you have an employee assistance programme that incorporates legal support during family court sagas? Is leadership (from the CEO to team managers) aware of what the family courts are like, so they can offer the flexibility your staff will need during this season?
- **Men (general):** Look out for your mates. If they're in the family courts, it's likely to consume them, draining them financially and emotionally, and after it all, they may not even come out of the process with the contact they wanted.
- **Dads (in the court process):** Keep your communication with your ex-partner squeaky clean at all times and regardless of what you have to endure. Do not vent on

social media. Polite and calm is the only way forward. You'll be glad you vented with your mates in the pub and deleted the angry email you were about to send. Even if your ex's communication is aggressive and outrageously unfair, do not join in or match it. Keep records of it, take screenshots, and respond calmly and politely. Save your aggression for the gym. Create a buddy system with wise and measured people and reach out to them first. In this scenario, a wise and measured person wouldn't encourage behaviour/action that might set you along a path of war in the family courts. Wise and measured people would see war as an absolute last resort. War is good for no one.

Understand that the court wheels turn painfully slowly. You can't speed them up. You have to play the game – it's not a nice game, but it works better for you if you stick to the rules.

Recognise that you're entering a tough period of your life, so reach out to your mates, participate in community, find outlets to help you manage the stress, but which don't ruin your finances or health.

If your contact is restricted, then bear in mind the words of Scott Mair in the 36th episode of *Men on Show*: 'There's a lot you can achieve in just 15–20 minutes of quality contact, so turn your phone off, switch off all other distractions and focus entirely on the child(ren) with games, attention, interaction.'

Dads and paternity leave

From one massive topic to another: paternity leave. If there's one thing we could do to benefit dads, mums and their children, it's address the UK's stingy paternity leave allowance for employed dads. It's probably the only thing that men's rights activists and militant feminists would agree on! At the point of writing this book, dads get up to two weeks' paternity leave allowance paid at either £187.18 each week, or 90 per cent of their earnings, whichever is lower. This is currently being reviewed by the UK government and no doubt on the very day this book is published and launched, the government will announce major changes to the provision!

But for now at least, at a time in his life when a man most needs to bring home the bacon and help provide for his family unit, while also looking after his partner and embracing a massive life change, in the UK working dads are entitled to paternity leave, but just two weeks, and in order to use this allowance, the family unit takes a big financial hit, because most dads' weekly wages will be significantly higher than £187.18 each week.

Maybe this doesn't sound too bad? Maybe it's better now than before? Maybe it's his choice to be a dad; we can't have everything in life, so let's stop complaining and just get on with it? Why should tax-paying people who are not parents be funding people who are? Outside the UK, things are a bit different for families in Western Europe. Rather than work through every country, I'll give you a snapshot of a few:

- **Spain:** 16 weeks, fully paid paternity leave.
- **Denmark:** Dads can take up to 24 weeks off work at full pay from the state (go Denmark!).
- **Poland:** Two weeks' fully paid leave, with an extra nine weeks of leave that can be taken if the parent is employed, at a rate of 70 per cent of the salary, and until the child is six years old.
- **Sweden:** *(For the British fathers reading this, you may want to sit down.)* Parents receive a whopping 480 days of paid parental leave per child. This can be shared between two parents (typically 240 days each) or taken in full by a single parent. There are 90 non-transferable days per parent,

with the remuneration for 390 days calculated at 80 per cent of your salary, before it reduces (Johnson 2025).

I spent hours berating myself for not being able to hold my shit together as a new dad, but in researching how other European countries provide for new employed parents and comparing it with the UK's pitiful provision, I now feel less inadequate.

Maybe you feel caught between delivering for your employer but knowing you're badly needed at home: it's something I struggled with mentally. Maybe you've put everything else on hold, because providing and childcare responsibilities has maxed you out. The reality is that your European cousins have it much better than you. Would you feel so burnt out as a working father if you had the Swedish model supporting you? Probably not! The three categories affecting paternal wellbeing that I mentioned earlier in this chapter (time bonding with the infant, confidence in your caring abilities and ability to provide) are achievable and in no way contradictory – but only if you're parenting within a system which takes parenting seriously.

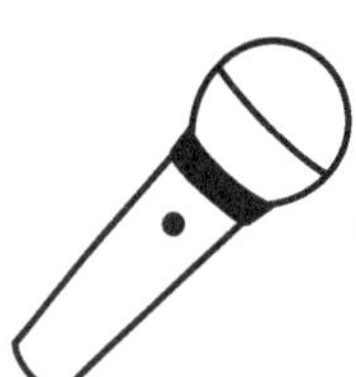

Jeremy Davies, *Men on Show*, episode 29

> Jeremy Davies is the CEO of the Fatherhood Institute and a major driver of his work is to increase the levels of paternity leave for dads in the UK. On the podcast, he referenced a phone-in show he was part of with LBC, where a caller, a professional chef, described his 12-hour shifts from 10.30 am to 10.30 pm, six days per week, leaving only one day of the week to see his kids. The chef expressed with great sadness that when he saw his kids, he didn't know how to be with them, because he saw so little of them.

The breadwinner's penalty: not something you'll read

about in the media, but when we think of working dads and 'privilege', often he's not a suited and booted executive, on the cusp of being a corporate top dog, enjoying first-class business trips to Milan with the cash pouring in. He's more likely to be a dad working a DAD (dirty and dangerous) job, as referenced in Chapter 1, a minimum wage job, or a role with little or no flexibility, no option for flexitime and no possibility of working from home. We've heard a lot about the motherhood penalty and so we should. We should also consider the implications of the male breadwinner's penalty.

A big step forward for supporting British men is better paternity leave in the UK, both in terms of the time available and also the financial support. It's something that might also contribute to closing the gender pay gap, given that the pay gap is driven almost entirely by parenting pressures. Major household names such as Deloitte, Aviva and John Lewis have equalised paternity leave in the UK as part of their employee offering. John Lewis, for example, offers 26 weeks of paid leave, with 14 weeks at full pay and 12 weeks at 50 per cent pay, available equally to all parents. It's great to see these brands taking the lead and no doubt others will follow, but for smaller organisations, charities and microenterprises, improving paternity leave will require government commitment and resources.

Based on calculations made by researchers at the University of Bath, the cost of extending paternity leave to six weeks at 90 per cent of average earnings is approximately £.5 billion annually (Clifton-Sprigg et al 2025). So the key question is: would six weeks of paid paternity leave deliver a long-term return on the half-billion-quid investment? It's a question that is difficult to answer for sure, but in the same research study, an estimated social return of £14 billion annually was suggested, and on my podcast with Jeremy Davies, he referenced research where 25 per cent of British voters said their vote would be influenced by where a political party stood on paternity leave.

How do you create an unbreakable bond with your children?

This third and final question of the chapter is one of my favourite topics. I'm no expert and I'm always learning. Sometimes I get it wrong, but based on countless conversations with other fathers, based on my lived experience (successes and failures) and wider research, there are four key points to deliver on as fathers. I'm not saying these alone will make you a fantastic father, but if finances are tight, you feel like you don't measure up and you think you're doing a lousy job as a dad, then deliver on these four things.

1. **Adventures and time:** Give them to your children. Be part of those adventures and share your time. On a recent all-inclusive holiday to Madeira, we stayed for 11 days in a fancy hotel. But what did our boys come back to the UK raving about? Adventures and quality time: finding awesome spots to jump into the sea from ever-increasing heights and dolphin-spotting from a speedboat. Those moments meant so much. Time was the other thing: the card games we played every evening before dinner – true magic! Dinner could have been less elaborate, they'd have been fine with a more modest hotel, but don't miss out on the card game or the adrenaline-filled jumps into the sea! If finances are tight for you (they were for me for years, not helped by two family court sagas), then focus on adventures and time: you don't need to go as far as Madeira for them, although I recommend it as a family holiday destination.

2. **Your child's setbacks, behavioural issues and lousy choices don't mean you're a lousy parent:** Your parenting style shapes your children to some extent, but if they're behind at school,

it's not necessarily a reflection of your parenting skills. If your neighbour's kids are polite and volunteer in worthy activities while your kids resent your every move, then rest assured, it's not your fault and you haven't failed. Your kid was already being shaped, long before they were born. Whether your kid wins or fails: it's not your fault. You're not a sculptor with mouldable clay. They are their own person. We can influence children to some extent and try to give them the best start in life, but we can't sculpt them into what we'd like them to be.

3. Get them used to expressing negative feelings so it becomes normal: When I meet suicide prevention trainers and campaigners through the course of my work, I often ask this important question: is there anything that parents can do today to reduce the chances of their children dying by suicide when they're older? The answer is generally the same: get them used to talking about negative feelings. For example, in my house, before bed, and on most nights (not all, but most) I have the chat with my boys, each one in turn. The conversation has evolved over time. When they were younger (under seven years old) I'd ask them to; a) tell me something that made them happy today; b) tell me something that made them sad today; and c) tell me something they're worried about. Sometimes they'd open up, and sometimes they'd make up trivial stuff (like being worried about their own farts), but it doesn't matter. The habit created a culture of talking openly and an acceptance that it's OK to feel worried or sad and say so. As they got older, the conversation changed and we moved to scoring the day, which sounds like this:

> Me: 'Out of 10, how would you rank today?' (10 being fantastic, 5 being moderate, 1 being dreadful)
> Him: 'About a 6.'
> Me: 'Six is good. How come it wasn't higher?' (And then follow up with, 'And why was it a 6 and not a 3?')

I still score the days with my thirteen- and ten-year-old, and have just started scoring with my seven-year-old. Scoring works well with adults too and can open up the conversation if you've asked your mate if he's OK, but you're not getting much back.

4. **Understand the science:** There's something that turns our fatherly world upside down: those teen years, they're not easy, and as dads, we can try to shrug it off or we can develop a rudimentary understanding of what's happening. During adolescence, your teen is undergoing serious brain development and one of the issues is that the amygdala, the brain's threat detector, becomes very sensitive (Vasa et al 2011). This is partly why your teen has a new and unwelcome tendency to 'fly off the handle' at perfectly reasonable requests.

Sadly, the frontal cortex, which drives long-term decision making, impulse control and understanding consequences, isn't yet developed and it won't fully develop until the early to mid-twenties (Arain et al 2013). To make things even worse, during adolescence, the resting baseline of dopamine is lower than in childhood or adulthood, which means teens are more likely to feel bored and need higher levels of both stimulation and risk in order to feel engaged (Wahlstrom et al 2011). Together, these changes can make teens volatile, dissatisfied and ungrateful for the things they have. Frankly, they won't give a shit about all you do for them day to day, nor your sacrifices in raising them from birth.

It's not that you shouldn't try to nurture responsible, decent adults who can stand on their own feet – of course you should. It's just that it's bloody hard and you'll have years of tearing your hair out in despair and frustration. If that's you right now, understand that what you're dealing with is troublesome brain development (which is a total pain in the arse), but your teen is not inherently rotten.

It's tough. I feel your pain. I previously said that Mother Nature knows best, but seriously, on teen brain development, what was she thinking?

As a dad, you are OK. You're doing the best you can. Most teens come out the other side, as will you.

Fatherhood: we've explored some massive topics in this chapter, from postnatal depression to the family courts, teenage brain development, the impact of both fatherlessness and parental alienation, and how to connect with your kids. I appreciate I've fired a lot of topics at you within the longest chapter in this book, but I hope that whether you're a biological father, a stepfather, legal guardian or concerned uncle or neighbour to a family with boys, you've taken something of value to help you in your role. To conclude the book, there is one key topic to finish with: the man code and how we think about masculinity.

10 Redefining masculinity

The stage was set. The pool was warm enough to get in (but not too warm). The lights were dimmed and strains of Mozart drifted through the air. An oasis of serenity had been created, an oasis which thankfully the kids couldn't ruin because they were staying with my parents. For my part, it was mission accomplished. Now that the midwife had arrived, the pressure was off... well, it was off me at least!

Henry is our third (and final) boy. He was making his transition from womb to world when the midwife's shift came to an end, but due to NHS protocols for home births, she couldn't leave our house until the next midwife arrived to take over. At the same time, the nitrous oxide gas had been ordered, so we were also expecting the motorcycle courier to arrive. The knock on my door at 11 pm was therefore fully expected. It was either the midwife or the NHS courier delivering the gas, and given the person on my doorstop was a bloke, it was clearly the gas. But strangely, the bloke was lacking motorcycle gear and even more strangely, he was wearing a midwifery uniform. Still believing him to be the courier (because he was a bloke), I asked if he had the gas, to which he replied that he was the midwife.

I was stunned. It's not that I felt weird about another bloke being present at a very intimate scene, but my mind was spinning. I only want the very best midwife for my wife and unborn child, and this guy cannot be the best... because he's a guy! Surely, he's in the wrong job? We have a long Edwardian terraced house and thankfully, by the time I'd followed him along the hallway and into the kitchen, I was rapidly pulling myself together. He was a brilliant midwife, a married man himself with a child of his own.

Gender bias: predefined views of what it is that a man or woman does, anticipating what he's likely to be good at or not, what his probable interests will be, how his character will form and how he might react to complexity, challenge and all manner of social interactions – his needs, preferences, demands. We make quick assumptions, all based on whether a person is a male or female. It's embarrassing that with so much information at our fingertips, we're still so impulsive, stupid and narrow minded. But gender bias is common: most of us are guilty of it, one way or the other. So, to conclude our honest exploration of what it is to be a man today, it seems fitting to end with a chapter on masculinity and whether we can redefine how we think about it. How do we think about masculinity so that it's:

- fit for the 21st century?
- a positive model for the next and current generation of men?
- *not* restrictive?

There are those who argue the very idea of 'redefining' masculinity is not helpful because it indicates that masculinity needs fixing, which it doesn't. But with so much conversation today about masculinity and whether the phrase toxic masculinity is helpful or in need of being binned, I think it's important to have a conversation about masculinity and what kind of men we want to be. I'm personally comfortable with the words 'redefine' and 'reimagine', so long as the conversation is positive, so long as it doesn't restrict masculinity to a rigid set of expectations and so long as we're conscious that what we're seeking to evolve is not masculinity itself, but our ideas about masculinity.

On the infamous *Joe Rogan Experience* podcast in January 2025, Mark Zuckerberg, founder, chairman and CEO of Meta Platforms, Inc (Facebook, WhatsApp, Instagram, etc) complained that corporate culture in America had been 'culturally neutered', moving away from 'masculine energy'. He was advocating for the celebration of aggression, arguing that masculinity has a positive side, that it's not all bad. He was quick to also point out that masculine energies shouldn't outweigh feminine energies, and a healthy environment would have a balance between both. At first glance, this seems reasonable. It's widely accepted that:

- **Masculine energies** = aggressive, dominant, competitive, decisive, action-orientated, autonomous.
- **Feminine energies** = compassionate, empathic, collaborative (the so-called softer elements of human traits).

But who gets to decide which of the above traits are more feminine or masculine?

Some of the most aggressive people I've ever had the misfortune to interact with include both men and women, and some of the most empathic and collaborative people I've ever met also include both men and women. Some thinkers would argue that those super-aggressive people I refer to (men and women) have their masculine/feminine balances out of kilter (as do those who are super-compliant).

- But would you seriously suggest to a woman that she needs more masculine energy? (Other than when she's asking for an overdue pay rise or going for promotion.)
- Or if she's a people pleaser and seeks harmony often at her own expense, would you honestly suggest to her that the answer lies in embracing masculine tendencies?

I'm guessing most of you wouldn't. You might suggest she needs better boundaries, but you're unlikely to encourage a woman to become more masculine. And when you have a man who is aggressive and dominant, would you try to influence his behaviour by encouraging him to become more feminine?

The words 'masculine' and 'feminine' are both so steeped in meaning (and possible misunderstanding) that what one person might imply from your use of these words could be very different from the next, and aside from misunderstanding, there is another *big* problem with these terms. If as men we accept the 'masculine'/'feminine' trait models, then many of the 'masculine' traits are reminiscent of a self-centred caveman, whereas the feminine traits are those of someone with higher levels of emotional intelligence. As a modern man, I find this description of masculine traits quite insulting to read, and if the essence of man is 'aggressive', 'dominant', 'competitive', then it's probably best to squash it and feminise all men. But if masculinity is squashed and men are put on a feminisation programme, you'll get what we're getting today: angry, disillusioned groups of men, who feel forgotten, lost and are moving to the right of the political spectrum (and women wondering where all the good men are!).

A brief history of masculine and feminine terms

Let's go back to the beginning. In simple terms, the constructs of masculinity and femininity were introduced by sociological scholars and researchers in the 20th century. They started to challenge the accepted narrative that sex-based behaviour was biologically determined, or in plain English, they started to challenge the belief that how men and women behave is driven by nature rather than nurture.

Within that context, researchers started categorising how

people conformed to the gendered expectations of society and in most cases, either you were the 'breadwinner' (male) or the 'homemaker' (female). The conversation has of course evolved through the 20th century as family and working structures have changed, and increasingly today, people are both breadwinners and homemakers. There are exceptions, of course. Some people win bread and try to keep the home stuff to a minimum. Some are homemakers first and foremost but do a bit of bread-winning through a side hustle. And, of course, there are a few people (men and women) who don't win bread or make good the home!

The majority of people today accept the mixing up of breadwinning and homemaking roles as part of modern society, but the traits that we still associate with the words 'masculine' and 'feminine' remain firmly stuck in 20th-century thinking. They've not yet caught up with societal shifts. In theory, at least, a trait should indicate how a person is likely to think, feel and act. Traits are supposed to be an enduring aspect of a particular person and at the core of their being (so not likely to change much or quickly). But there are a few issues with categorising traits into either a masculine or feminine camp.

1. Context matters. People don't always act according to their traits. A person seen as aggressive will not be aggressive in every situation. In some situations, they might be more placid than an easy-going person and 'aggressive people' may experience life events that either reduce or increase their aggressive tendencies.
2. When we define people in terms of a small set of traits, putting them in one camp or another, we don't allow for the rich diversity and complexity of people.
3. Your version of masculinity traits may be very different from my version, so who's wrong and who's right? Can we both be right?

4. What about those people who may not see themselves as a man or woman, or they've transitioned from one to the other?

So, the question remains: how do we redefine our ideas about masculinity in a meaningful, inclusive, positive and non-patronising way, so that we can create something that inspires the current and next generation of men, and so that we can replace the dreadful toxic masculinity language and all that is associated with it?

We could give masculinity a rebrand and talk about positive masculinity, flexible masculinity or maybe the gentleman's code. Or maybe we just need to embrace our inbuilt, 'Liver King' personality (but without the performance-enhancing drugs – see Chapter 5). There's no easy answer, but in talking about masculinity with boys and men, I recommend four points to consider as conversation starters.

It's nature *and* nurture

Girls and boys, women and men: we're different, we're unpredictable (because we're human), and neither gender is more prone to being toxic than the other. I've raised two daughters (who are now in their early twenties) and three sons (who are still growing up – aged seven, ten and 13), and having raised both genders, their behavioural differences never fail to astound me. I appreciate that five children from one family unit is a limited sample size, but as young children, my daughters could sit calmly at the table for a meal, wait until everyone had finished and have a respectful conversation. At times, they would argue and fight as most siblings do, but there was always a logical reason that could be identified for the argument, even if the reason itself was trivial.

If my daughters didn't get out of the house on a weekend morning, then no problem, they could absorb themselves in craft activities, Playmobil or Lego, creating community-based play such as hospitals, holidays and family life. As long as they got outside at some point in the day, morning or afternoon, then parenting them, as young children at least, was pretty straightforward (it got tougher when they became teens).

And my boys? They play with Lego and Playmobil as their sisters did, but games will generally have warfare at their heart. We limit their access to toy weapons, but I don't know why we bother, because they just make weapons out of whatever they can find. Only last year, my then eight-year-old asked Santa for a meat cleaver and a sword. He felt it was a reasonable request, given they would be used for his *Lord of the Rings* battle re-enactments! My daughters have literally never had weapons on their Santa wish lists.

My boys can't leave each other alone. From wake-up to bedtime, they'll play-fight, again and again. It *always* starts in play, and it *always* ends in tears. As for sitting still at the table for a meal and respectful conversation, *forget that*: our meals are like feeding time at the zoo. If any of them have used the cutlery at any point during the meal, I feel I've succeeded that day as a parent. At weekends, if we don't get the boys out of the house by 10 am, it's utter chaos and the house is turned upside down.

Is it nature or nurture? You'll meet die-hard believers from both camps. Some will insist my sons and daughters have hardwiring that explains my parenting challenges. Others will say it's down to society, education, my parenting approach and the media. The science seems pretty clear, though, that from the impact of elevated testosterone in men's bodies (which particularly peaks when boys go through puberty), through to the pace and nature of infant brain development, men and women are built a bit differently and while there are always exceptions to the rule, it's OK to conclude that, typically, most men would be more likely to demonstrate a particular behaviour or preference in a certain context, and women in another. It's OK to conclude this – as long as we also accept that these are 'probables' not 'set in stone'.

And it's also OK to conclude that added to biological differences, parents, media and society may unwittingly give signals and messages that impact how a man, woman, person may develop, how they may feel about who they are and what they perceive they're capable of. If we can accept both things, then let's get comfy with initiatives that might be more geared towards women's common tendencies, and initiatives that might be more geared towards men's common tendencies, understanding that no preference or tendency is fixed: they're driven by nature and nurture, and unravelling which 'n' played a more influential role in shaping you will have you plummeting down rabbit holes from which there'll be no return.

Celebrate masculinity

I've mentioned this before in Chapter 4. From the Carnegie Award heroes to the Thai cave rescue and my podcast, male heroes are everywhere, but we don't hear much about them. So, who should we look to for inspiration? Who should the next generation hold as their role models? Where are the positive man codes that we can reflect on, to maximise our potential?

Caitlin Moran is an English journalist and broadcaster and in her best-selling book, *What About Men?* (2023), she makes the point that generally, when we see men in the news, it's because he murdered someone or invaded a country, but when it comes to a 'top 10 men who are changing the world' list, or 'the 20 most inspiring men from 2025' or 'the 101 inspiring boys from history' book, there's been a glaring silence where there needs to be noise and energy. It's that 'gamma bias' phenomenon I mentioned in Chapter 4!

Moran goes further, to list the favourite behavioural patterns she's experienced from the men in her life, including:

- less judgemental, with less backstabbing or bitchy comments; more protective of those they love
- up for an adventure (even daft initiatives destined to fail, such as snowboarding the tea-tray down the stairs)
- hard working (particularly on outdoor and manual tasks)
- joyful and full of banter
- practical tinkerers with a fascination for how things work
- a huge urge to be helpful and swoop in.

It's not that women don't demonstrate these traits – and these are Moran's reflections based on her own experiences, rather than global research – but they make their own point. For all the horrible stuff in the news perpetrated by men, for all the talk about misogyny and toxic masculinity, at their core, the vast majority of men are wonderful, kind, loyal and want to create a better world. At their core, men typically may also have leanings towards certain skills and behaviours. Being proactive about celebrating them (without the caveat of 'we need to also recognise the part his male privilege played in getting him to this point') is an important step forward in forging a healthier perspective of who we can be and what we can become. It's the reason I started my podcast. It's the reason I continue it.

Avoiding the prescribed approach

My man code is personal to me, so while the question of how we redefine masculinity is an important conversation to be having, I don't want to impose my version of masculinity on other men. I could add a PhD on gender studies to my CV, an MSc, MBE, diploma or anything else I fancy, but they still wouldn't give my version of masculinity an edge over yours. If we want to nurture rounded and healthy men, if we want to see men enjoying being men, leaning into masculinity, then we need to accept that masculinity is broad and varied, not narrow and predictable; it's grey rather than black and white. We should be having open conversations about our man codes, laughing together, respectfully challenging each other and reflecting on the men we want to be.

Mike Nicholson was my 19th guest on *Men on Show*. He is a heavyweight figure (metaphorically speaking) in the boys and education arena and the organisation he founded and leads, Progressive Masculinity, works with boys in schools to help them think about masculinity in a safe and open setting, where they get to decide what kind of boyfriends, future lovers, dads and men they want to be. A former English teacher, he realised that many boys had behavioural issues because they believed that they needed to act in a certain way to gain respect, and their 'respect gaining' behaviour was negatively impacting their education and wellbeing. Mike decided to do something about this problem and got started, trialling masculinity sessions with boys in his own school before founding Progressive Masculinity.

Progressive Masculinity works intensively with the 12 most influential boys, as identified by the school, over a two-day period. They explore topics such as healthy relationships, banter, body image, masculinity and the digital world, and emotional communication, and give the boys space to reflect and form their own views about these topics. The boys become masculinity ambassadors and are tasked with changing the culture at the school from within, working in many cases as peer mentors and helping teachers to shape the PHSE lessons.

At no point do Mike and the team impose their view of masculinity on the boys: it's about creating a safe space, enabling the boys to open up and talk about their values (the three most commonly cited by boys being resilience, selflessness and loyalty) as well as develop their critical thinking skills, so when they're surfing the web at home and jumping from one social media platform to the other, they're equipped to ask better questions about what they're consuming.

Does the work of Progressive Masculinity sound like a more intelligent approach for developing the next generation of men, rather than teams going into schools to tackle the scourge of toxic masculinity?

It does to me!

What is true for boys is also true for us men. In a world of quick headlines and increasing polarisation, there is an urgent need for safe spaces and critical thinking, so we can think about what kind of men we want to be and form our own opinions, but without the bravado, and with our masks fully off. And in order to create psychologically safe spaces for men, we need psychological safety, and we need men's communities (the topics of Chapters 7 and 8).

Open minds

Daniele Fiandaca, my 43rd podcast guest, has built his work today around male allyship in the workplace and challenging traditional stereotypes around masculinity. He founded the Hard as Nails programme, celebrating men painting their nails, and he's been training as a nail technician to run his own nail bar. I asked him why he does it. It intrigued me: does he paint his nails because he wants to? Or to make a statement?

Daniele explained that he was inspired by his friend who painted his nails because his daughter had asked him to in preparation for a Harry Styles concert (Harry Styles paints his nails). But after the concert, his friend couldn't take the nail paint off for about a week because it was shellac, and so he was stuck with the painted nails, something which prompted lots of nail/men/masculinity conversations that particular week.

Daniele's aim in painting his nails and encouraging guys to do the same is to create a catalyst for wider conversation around masculinity, exploring the man-code stereotypes and embracing a version of masculinity that is much broader and inclusive. As a result of the nail painting, he's also found new ways to connect with his nieces and goddaughters. His choices have not always been welcomed from wider society. Daniele occasionally wears skirts and his wife works for Childline, so in support of his wife's employer, Daniele attended a Pride march in London, wearing a Childline T-shirt matched with a skirt. Within a day, he was being branded a paedophile on social media. It's why we need to raise a generation of sound and open-minded critical thinkers.

- Who says that men can't wear skirts or paint their nails?
- Who says that having pink-dyed hair makes any kind of statement about your sexuality?
- Who says that personal grooming is for sissies and not for real men (whatever a real man is)?

Would I paint my nails? Probably not. It just doesn't interest me – I'm colour blind and tend to leave colouring decisions to my wife, who isn't colour blind. My personal interests involve my chin-up bar, diving (off diving boards), playing football, running, pubs and restaurants, none of which make me more or less manly than the next guy. It's just what I'm into. And alongside my interests, if I'm watching an emotionally charged movie, even if it's just soppy nonsense, I'll be the first to cry, long before my wife! Just to clarify that: when emotionally charged movies are on the screen, chin-up bar Pain is the most likely tear-spiller in our home!

The more we can be open about masculinity as a broad, endless and positive concept, rather than a narrow and prone-to-being-toxic one, the better for everyone's mental health. Let's not forget that those pesky Vikings who instilled terror in communities along the English coast may have killed and plundered at will, but on the other hand, they rather liked their grooming days and valued cleanliness. In Old Norse, Saturday was *Laugardagr* (bath day) with archaeological digs finding combs, tweezers and washing gear!

As men, let's foster open minds that say 'Why not?' and 'Go for it' to the boys who are interested in studying midwifery. Let's say 'Why not?' and 'Go for it' to the lads who want to paint their nails one week at school (either because they just want to, or because they want to start conversations about masculinity). Let's say 'Why not?' and 'Go for it' to men who claim collaboration, empathy and harmony as their core masculine traits. I'm not arguing with it. Are you?

Andy's man code

My man code has evolved over the years because I've taken time to think about what kind of man I aspire to be and where my rigid guidelines on how to be a good man have let me down, from my drive to be a knight in shining armour, rescuing damsels in distress, to the pressure of being *the* provider and *the* protector, which is OK if you're feeling confident and you're happily employed with healthy finances, but when you're unemployed with a bleak financial future, it's truly crushing.

Today for example, I am a contributor and people developer. I want to help other people be their best, and that passion is channelled as much towards men, people, women, rather than simply damsels in distress. I'm now as likely to give my seat on the train for an elderly man as I am an elderly woman. I see myself as *a* protector not *the* protector. In fact, when it comes to protecting my children online, my wife takes the lead as she's far more tech savvy than me. And I'm *a* provider, but not *the* provider, understanding that provision comes in many forms, not just hard cash. We can 'provide' through the giving of our time, focus, experience and skills, through positive role modelling and mentoring the next generation of people.

- What does your man code look like?
- Is it fit for purpose? Or does it let you down?
- How will you evolve your man code over the next three months?

Psychological safety, men's communities, fatherhood and redefining masculinity – in these topics we find the answers to creating better outcomes for men. Not all the answers, I hasten to add, and of course there are more answers woven into the chapters in Part 1 of the book.

I fully appreciate that it's not possible to cover every conceivable angle on helping men to be their best in one book, but there is an army of people taking pen to paper, fingers to laptops, faces to video cameras, and creating valuable resources to help reduce gender division and improve the outcomes for men, women and people. It's an honour to be part of that army.

Thanks for investing your time in reading this book and thanks again for buying it. Your purchase has been good news for the men's and boys' grassroots projects in need of funding!

References

Adams, R (2025) 'Barking at female staff and blocking doorways: Teachers warn of rise in misogyny and racism in UK schools'. *The Guardian* 19 April. URL: theguardian.com/education/2025/apr/19/teachers-warn-rise-misogyny-racism-uk-schools

Advance HE (2025) 'Governance news alert: HESA enrolment data 2023/24. URL: advance-he.ac.uk/knowledge-hub/governance-news-alert-hesa-enrolment-data-202324

Alvarez-Garcia, P, Garcia-Fernandez, R et al (2024) 'Postpartum depression in fathers: A systematic review'. National Library of Medicine 16 May. URL: pmc.ncbi.nlm.nih.gov/articles/PMC11122550

American Psychological Association (2022) 'Stress in America 2022: Concerned for the future, beset by inflation'. October. URL: apa.org/news/press/releases/stress/2022/concerned-future-inflation

Arain, M, Haque, M et al (2013) 'Maturation of the adolescent brain'. National Library of Medicine 3 April. URL: pmc.ncbi.nlm.nih.gov/articles/PMC3621648

BACP (2025) 'Men's attitudes to counselling and how they differ to women's'. 11 June. URL: bacp.co.uk/news/news-from-bacp/2025/9-june-men-s-attitudes-to-therapy-and-how-they-differ-to-women-s

Bamishigbin Jr, O N, Wilson, D K et al (2020) 'Father involvement in infant parenting in an ethnically diverse community sample: Predicting paternal depressive symptoms'. Frontiers in Psychiatry, 23 September. URL: frontiersin.org/journals/psychiatry/articles/10.3389/fpsyt.2020.578688/full

Bancroft, H (2025) 'More than a third of young men who watch masculinity influencers act on their advice, research finds'. *The Independent* 23 April. URL: independent.co.uk/news/uk/home-news/social-media-masculinity-men-andrew-tate-b2737180.html

BBC Food (2019) 'What is ultra-processed food and what does it mean for my health?' URL: bbc.co.uk/food/articles/what_is_ultra-processed_food

BBC News (2009) 'Fathers-to-be "gain extra weight"'. 22 May. URL: news.bbc.co.uk/1/mobile/health/8063004.stm

Beal, J & Smart, Y (2024) 'The nation's birthrate has plummeted. How did we get here?' *The Times* 28 October. URL: thetimes.com/uk/society/article/the-nations-birthrate-has-plummeted-how-did-we-get-here-30qtqddwn

Berardelli, I & Rogante, E et al (2022) 'Is lethality different between males and females? Clinical and gender differences in inpatient suicide attempters'. National Library of Medicine. 15 October. URL: pmc.ncbi.nlm.nih.gov/articles/PMC9602518

Block, I (2024) 'Are you 'mankeeping'? How women are bearing the brunt of the male loneliness epidemic'. *The Standard* 6 November. URL: standard.co.uk/lifestyle/mankeeping-male-loneliness-women-invisible-labour-b1189365.html

Borysenko, K (2020) ' The dark side of #MeToo: What happens when men are falsely accused'. *Forbes* 12 February. URL: forbes.com/sites/karlynborysenko/2020/02/12/the-dark-side-of-metoo-what-happens-when-men-are-falsely-accused

Brader, C (2024) 'In focus: Housing needs of young people'. House of Lords Library 7 March. URL: lordslibrary.parliament.uk/housing-needs-of-young-people

Bratsberg, B, Kotsadam, A & Walther, S (2021) 'Male fertility: Facts, distribution and drivers of inequality'. IZA Discussion Papers No. 14506, provided in cooperation with IZA (Institute of Labor Economics). URL: econstor.eu/bitstream/10419/245557/1/dp14506.pdf

Bryant, M (2024) 'The Finnish miracle: How the country halved its suicide rate – and saved countless lives'. *The Guardian*. 22 October. URL: theguardian.com/world/2024/feb/22/the-finnish-miracle-how-the-country-halved-its-suicide-rate-and-saved-countless-lives

Business Rescue Expert (2025) 'As half of the UK's nightclubs shut for good – does this mean the party's over?' URL: businessrescueexpert.co.uk/as-half-of-the-uks-nightclubs-shut-for-good-does-this-mean-the-partys-over

Butt, M (2025) 'Marcus Brigstocke opens up about "shameful" and "lonely" porn addiction'. *The Independent* 29 January. URL: independent.co.uk/arts-entertainment/comedy/news/marcus-brigstocke-porn-addiction-b2688116.html

Cappelen A W, Falch, R & Tungodden, B (2025) 'Experimental evidence on the acceptance of males falling behind'. *Journal of the European Economic Association*, 12 April. URL: academic.oup.com/jeea/advance-article/doi/10.1093/jeea/jvaf016/8112864

Cardiff University (2022) 'People from England's most deprived areas ten times more likely to be in prison, analysis finds'. 16 November. URL: cardiff.ac.uk/news/view/2684824-people-from-englands-most-deprived-areas-ten-times-more-likely-to-be-in-prison,-analysis-finds

Carnegie Hero Fund: carnegieherofundtrust.org

Carr, C (2024) 'Let's stop telling teen boys they are toxic'. American Institute for Boys and Men 11 July. URL: aibm.org/commentary/lets-stop-telling-teen-boys-they-are-toxic/

Cassino, D (2024) 'FDU poll finds online betting leads to problems for young men'. Fairleigh Dickinson University 20 August. URL: fdu.edu/news/fdu-poll-finds-online-betting-leads-to-problems-for-young-men/?

Centre for Social Justice (2025) 'Lost Boys, State of the Nation'. URL: centreforsocialjustice.org.uk/wp-content/uploads/2025/03/CSJ-The_Lost_Boys.pdf

Children's Commissioner for England (2023) 'Evidence on pornography's influence on harmful sexual behaviour among children'. 9 May. URL: childrenscommissioner.gov.uk/resource/pornography-and-harmful-sexual-behaviour

Chodick, G, Epstein, S & Shalev, V (2020) 'Secular trends in testosterone – findings from a large state-mandate care provider'. National Library of Medicine 9 March. URL: pubmed.ncbi.nlm.nih.gov/32151259

Ciar, V, Polat, Y et al (2011) 'Effects of magnesium supplementation on testosterone levels of athletes and sedentary subjects at rest and after exhaustion'. National Library of Medicine April. URL: pubmed.ncbi.nlm.nih.gov/20352370

Clark, D (2025) 'Number and percentage of young adults living with their parents UK 1996-2024. Statista 10 September. URL: statista.com/statistics/285339/percentage-of-young-adults-living-with-parents-uk

Clement-Webb, E (2024) 'Sextortion: A growing threat targeting minors'. FBI Memphis 23 January. URL: fbi.gov/contact-us/field-offices/nashville/news/sextortion-a-growing-threat-targeting-minors

Clifton-Sprigg, J, Hunt A et al (2025) 'Costs and benefits of improved leave for fathers in the first year: Too good to ignore'. University of Bath policy brief June. URL: bath.ac.uk/publications/costs-and-benefits-of-improved-leave-for-fathers-in-the-first-year-too-good-to-ignore/attachments/costs-and-benefits-of-improved-leave-for-fathers.pdf

Coffey, H (2024) 'A "lonely deaths" epidemic is sweeping the UK as thousands go undiscovered for a week or more'. *The Independent* 8 July. URL: independent.co.uk/life-style/die-alone-lonely-death-b2573819.html

Cominetti, N & Costa, R et al (2022) 'Changing jobs? Change in the UK labour market and the role of worker mobility'. The Economy 2030 Inquiry. URL: economy2030.resolutionfoundation.org/wp-content/uploads/2022/01/Changing-jobs.pdf

Cox, D A (2021) 'American men suffer a friendship recession'. Survey Center on American Life 6 July. URL: americansurveycenter.org/commentary/american-men-suffer-a-friendship-recession

Cox, J (2025) 'Can millennial dads have it all? Millennial dads want to split parenting equally. They're still struggling to break the breadwinner stereotype'. *Business Insider* 9 July. URL: businessinsider.com/millennial-dads-paradox-coparenting-breadwinner-office-home-2025-7

Dattani, S (2025) 'Women live longer than men, but how much longer varies widely around the world'. Our World in Data. URL: ourworldindata.org/data-insights/women-live-longer-than-men-but-how-much-longer-varies-widely-around-the-world

Department for Education (2025) 'Autumn Term 2024/25: Suspensions and permanent exclusions in England'. Gov.uk. URL: explore-education-statistics.service.gov.uk/find-statistics/suspensions-and-permanent-exclusions-in-england

Department of Health & Social Care (2022) 'New review launched into vitamin D intake to help tackle health disparities'. 3 April. URL: gov.uk/government/news/new-review-launched-into-vitamin-d-intake-to-help-tackle-health-disparities

Department of Health & Social Care (2025) 'Men's health: A strategic vision for England'. 19 November. URL: assets.publishing.service.gov.uk/media/69400f3b5cc812f50aa421df/mens-health-a-strategic-vision-for-england.pdf

Devi, S, Saxena, J et al (2014) 'Effect of short-term physical exercise on serum total testosterone levels in young adults'. National Library of Medicine April-June. URL: pubmed.ncbi.nlm.nih.gov/25509972

Diabetes.co.uk (2016) 'Men experience an abrupt decrease in testosterone levels after sugar intake, study finds'. 19 September. URL: diabetes.co.uk/news/2016/

sep/men-experience-an-abrupt-decrease-in-testosterone-levels-after-sugar-intake,-study-finds-99746064.html
Diaz, C, Rezende, L F M et al (2023) 'Artificially sweetened beverages and health outcomes: An umbrella review'. Science Direct, *Advances in Nutrition*. Vol 14 issue 4, July. URL: sciencedirect.com/science/article/pii/S2161831323003150
Dixon, S J (2025) 'Distribution of Tinder monthly active users in the United States as of March 2021'. Statista 19 August. URL: statista.com/statistics/975925/us-tinder-user-ratio-gender
Dizik, A (2024) 'More dads are taking parental leave than ever. Moms aren't always happy about it'. *The Guardian*. 16 February. URL: theguardian.com/lifeandstyle/2024/feb/16/paternity-maternity-leave-unequal
Dokoupil, T & Finn, N (2023) 'Millions of men have dropped out of the workforce, leaving companies struggling to fill jobs: It's "a matter of our national identity"'. *CBS News* 26 January. URL: cbsnews.com/news/men-workforce-work-companies-struggle-fill-jobs-manufacturing
Dolan, E W (2023) 'Having a negative perception of masculinity is linked to worse mental health'. *PsyPost* 17 November. URL: psypost.org/having-a-negative-perception-of-masculinity-is-linked-to-worse-mental-health-study-finds/
Dugan, E & Crerar, P (2024) 'Harm from problem gambling in Great Britain "may be eight times higher than thought"'. *The Guardian*. 25 July. URL: theguardian.com/society/article/2024/jul/25/harm-from-problem-gambling-in-uk-may-be-eight-times-higher-than-thought-research-finds
Eisenegger, C, Haushofer, J & Fehr, E (2011) 'The role of testosterone in social interaction'. *Trends in Cognitive Sciences* 15(6). URL: haushofer.ne.su.se/publications/Eisenegger_et_al_TiCS_2011.pdf
Elsesser, K (2019) '60% of male managers are uncomfortable in job-related activities with women – here's why'. *Fortune* 17 May. URL: forbes.com/sites/kimelsesser/2019/05/17/60-of-male-managers-are-uncomfortable-in-job-related-activities-with-women-heres-why
Equimundo (2025) 'Report launch: State of American Men 2025 – economic anxiety is the new masculinity crisis'. URL: equimundo.org/report-launch-state-of-american-men-2025-economic-anxiety-is-the-new-masculinity-crisis
European Business Magazine (2024) 'How much is the global gambling industry worth?' 23 April. URL: europeanbusinessmagazine.com/business/how-much-is-the-global-gambling-industry-worth
European Environment Agency (2022) 'Who benefits from nature in cities? Social inequalities in access to urban green and blue spaces across Europe'. 1 February. URL: eea.europa.eu/en/analysis/publications/who-benefits-from-nature-in-cities-social-inequalities-in-access-to-urban-green-and-blue-spaces-across-europe
Families Outside (2023) 'Child poverty and the impact of imprisonment'. The Poverty Alliance. 9 October. URL: povertyalliance.org/guest-blog-child-poverty-and-the-impact-of-imprisonment/
Fenney, D & Raleigh, V (2024) 'Inequalities in men's health: Why are they not being addressed?' The King's Fund 12 June. URL: kingsfund.org.uk/insight-and-analysis/blogs/inequalities-mens-health-why-are-they-not-being-addressed
Foster, J (2022) 'Normal male testosterone levels'. Optimale 25 January. URL: optimale.co.uk/articles/normal-male-testosterone-levels
Glass, A (2024) 'London sees annual drop in community spaces with Brent hit

hardest'. Foundation for Future London 7 June. URL: future.london/article/london-sees-annual-drop-in-community-spaces-with-brent-hit-hardest

Goodale, T, Sadhu P et al (2017) 'Testosterone and the heart'. National Library of Medicine. April-June. URL: pmc.ncbi.nlm.nih.gov/articles/PMC5512682/

Graff, M (2017) 'Improving your chances on Tinder: Three research-based ways to improve your Tinder chances'. *Psychology Today*, 22 November. URL: psychologytoday.com/us/blog/love-digitally/201711/improving-your-chances-on-tinder

Graso, K & Reynolds, T (2024) 'A feminine advantage in the domain of harm: a review and path forward'. The Royal Society Publishing *Biology Letters* 13 November. URL: royalsocietypublishing.org/doi/10.1098/rsbl.2024.0381

Government Equalities Office, Women and Equalities Unit (2021) 'Shared care: fathers' involvement in care and family well-being outcomes: a literature review'. 15 January. URL: gov.uk/government/publications/childcare-shared-care-and-well-being-outcomes-for-families/shared-care-fathers-involvement-in-care-and-family-well-being-outcomes-a-literature-review?

Hanley, J & Williams, M (2020) 'Fathers' perinatal mental health'. *British Journal of Midwifery* 28(2).

Harding, A (2007) 'Men's testosterone levels declined in last 20 years'. Reuters. 9 August. URL: reuters.com/article/business/healthcare-pharmaceuticals/mens-testosterone-levels-declined-in-last-20-years-idUSKIM169763

Harman, J J, Leder-Elder, S & Biringen, Z (2019) 'Prevalence of adults who are the targets of parental alienating behaviors and their impact'. *Children and Youth Services Review*, Volume 106, November. URL: sciencedirect.com/science/article/abs/pii/S0190740919306164

Health and Safety Executive (2025) 'Work-related fatal injuries in Great Britain'. URL: hse.gov.uk/statistics/fatals-overview.htm

Heubeck, E (2025) 'Why school isn't working for many boys and what could help'. *Education Week*, 27 January. URL: edweek.org/leadership/why-school-isnt-working-for-many-boys-and-what-could-help/2025/01

Hine, B, Shaljean, S & Shaljean, J (2022) 'Teachers' experiences of the impact of fatherlessness on male pupils'. Lads Need Dads and University of West London research project. URL: ladsneeddads.org/wp-content/uploads/2024/06/2024-LND_-Report_Teachers-experiences-impact-2022.pdf

Hooven, C (2021) *Testosterone: The story of the hormone that dominates and divides us.* Cassell.

House of Commons Library (2025) 'Women and the UK economy, Research Briefing'. 28 February. URL: commonslibrary.parliament.uk/research-briefings/sn06838

Huaxia (2024) 'Japan sees over 37,000 people die alone at home in H1'. Xinhua.net 29 August. URL: english.news.cn/20240829/4f7f4e4778e84574921fff5e8acd1da9/c.html

Hughes, A (2024) 'The great "only child" myth: Why having no siblings will soon be a huge advantage'. BBC Science Focus 24 May. URL: sciencefocus.com/science/only-children

Hurst, K (2024) 'U.S. women are outpacing men in college completion, including in every major racial and ethnic group'. Pew Research Center, 18 November. URL: pewresearch.org/short-reads/2024/11/18/us-women-are-outpacing-men-in-college-completion-including-in-every-major-racial-and-ethnic-group

Internet Watch Foundation (2024) 'Teenage boys targeted as hotline sees "heartbreaking" increase in child "sextortion" reports'. 18 March. URL: iwf.org.uk/news-media/news/teenage-boys-targeted-as-hotline-sees-heartbreaking-increase-in-child-sextortion-reports

Johnson, K (2025) 'Paternity leave: How much time off work do new dads get across Europe?'. BBC News. 15 June. URL: bbc.co.uk/news/articles/cy8d3l7858zo

Kahl, K L (2020) 'Testosterone levels show steady decrease among young US men'. *Urology Times*, Yale School of Medicine. 3 July. URL: urologytimes.com/view/testosterone-levels-show-steady-decrease-among-young-us-men

Kim, P & Swain, J E (2007) 'Sad dads: Paternal postpartum depression'. National Library of Medicine 4 February. URL: pmc.ncbi.nlm.nih.gov/articles/PMC2922346

King, B M (2022) 'Does marrying younger mean marrying more often? When and how often people marry changes by birth cohort'. United States Census Bureau 31 August. URL: census.gov/library/stories/2022/08/does-marrying-younger-mean-marrying-more-often.html

Kirk-Wade, E (2025) 'Suicide statistics'. House of Commons Library, 8 January. URL: commonslibrary.parliament.uk/research-briefings/cbp-7749/

Kirk, I (2022) 'How often do Britons watch porn?' YouGov 1 July. URL: yougov.co.uk/society/articles/42945-how-often-do-britons-watch-porn

Koessl, G (2025) 'Home sweet hurdle'. IPS, Economy and Ecology, 24 March. URL: ips-journal.eu/topics/economy-and-ecology/home-sweet-hurdle-8180

Kumagai, H, Zempo-Miyaki, A et al (2015) 'Increased physical activity has a greater effect than reduced energy intake on lifestyle modification-induced increases in testosterone'. National Library of Medicine 27 November. URL: pmc.ncbi.nlm.nih.gov/articles/PMC4706091

Kumar, N (2025) 'Tinder statistics 2025 (users, revenue & demographics)'. *Demand Sage* 19 September. URL: demandsage.com/tinder-statistics

Lee, J (2025) 'More men in their prime working years are neither working nor looking for jobs – here's why'. *CNBC* 19 September. URL: cnbc.com/2024/09/21/why-more-men-are-dropping-out-of-the-workforce.html

Leproult, R & Van Cauter, E (2011) 'Effect of 1 Week of Sleep Restriction on Testosterone Levels in Young Healthy Men'. National Library of Medicine 1 June. URL: pmc.ncbi.nlm.nih.gov/articles/PMC4445839

Liu A, Akimova, E T et al (2024) 'Evidence from Finland and Sweden on the relationship between early-life diseases and lifetime childlessness in men and women' *Nature Human Behaviour* 8(2). URL: pubmed.ncbi.nlm.nih.gov/38110509

Lynch, P & Forsyth, A (2025) 'Schools, care homes and sports clubs sold off to pay spiralling council debt'. *BBC News* 26 August. URL: bbc.co.uk/news/articles/cq87497v8ypo

Mantua, J, Naylor, J A et al (2020) 'Sleep loss during military training reduces testosterone in U.S. Army Rangers: A two-study series'. Clin Med International Library. URL: clinmedjournals.org/articles/ijsem/international-journal-of-sports-and-exercise-medicine-ijsem-6-169.php

Martin, A J (2018)' "Winning" contests gives men testosterone boost, study suggests'. Sky News 9 August. URL: news.sky.com/story/winning-contests-gives-men-testosterone-boost-study-suggests-11465370

Mental Health UK (2025) 'Burnout Report 2025 reveals generational divide in levels of stress and work absence.' 16 January. URL: mentalhealth-uk.org/blog/

burnout-report-2025-reveals-generational-divide-in-levels-of-stress-and-work-absence/

Merlio (2025) 'Porn statistics 2024: Consumption data, demographics & global trends'. URL: merlio.app/blog/porn-statistics-2024-analysis-trends

Miller, R (2025) 'Men with paternal postnatal depression require better support'. Centre for Policy Research on Men and Boys. URL: menandboys.org.uk/nce/paternal-postnatal25

Ministry of Justice (2024) 'Family court statistics quarterly: October to December 2024'. URL: gov.uk/government/statistics/family-court-statistics-quarterly-october-to-december-2024

Ministry of Justice (2025) 'Offender employment outcomes – statistical summary'. Gov.uk 17 February. URL: gov.uk/government/statistics/offender-employment-outcomes-update-to-march-2024/offender-employment-outcomes-statistical-summary

Monson, N R, Klair, N et al (2023) 'Association between vitamin D deficiency and testosterone levels in adult males: A systematic review.' National Library of Medicine 24 September. URL: pmc.ncbi.nlm.nih.gov/articles/PMC10518189

Moosazadeh, M, Heydari, K et al (2024) 'Association of the effect of alcohol consumption on luteinizing hormone (LH), follicle-stimulating hormone (FSH), and testosterone hormones in men: A systematic review and meta-analysis'. National Library of Medicine 26 December. URL: pubmed.ncbi.nlm.nih.gov/39867254

Moran, C (2023) *What About Men?* Ebury Press.

Moran, R (2024) 'Girls outperform boys from primary school to university'. Cambridge University Press & Assessment. URL: cambridge.org/news-and-insights/girls-outperform-boys

Moreira, D, Azeredo, A & Dias, P (2023) 'Risk factors for gambling disorder: A Systematic Review'. National Library of Medicine 8 March. URL: pmc.ncbi.nlm.nih.gov/articles/PMC9994414

Movember Report (2024) 'The real face of men's health'. URL: uk.movember.com/movember-institute/the-real-face-of-mens-health-report

Ng, K (2022) 'Caring for grandchildren can fight off loneliness, study suggests'. *The Independent*, 24 November. URL: independent.co.uk/life-style/health-and-families/grandchildren-grandparents-care-loneliness-b2232048.html

Nordal, E (2020) 'Testosterone levels decreasing in Danish men'. *IceNews* 17 May. URL: icenews.is/2010/05/17/testosterone-levels-decreasing-in-danish-men/

OECD Affordable Housing Database, Social Policy Division, Directorate of Employment, Labour and Social Affairs (2023). 'Population experiencing homelessness. URL: oecd.org/content/dam/oecd/en/data/datasets/affordable-housing-database/hc3-1-homeless-population.pdf

Ofsted & His Majesty's Inspectorate of Prisons (2022) 'Prison education: A review of reading education in prisons'. Gov.uk 22 March. URL: gov.uk/government/publications/prison-education-a-review-of-reading-education-in-prisons/prison-education-a-review-of-reading-education-in-prisons

ONS (2022) 'Health state life expectancies by national deprivation deciles, England: 2018 to 2020'. URL: ons.gov.uk/peoplepopulationandcommunity/healthandsocialcare/healthinequalities/bulletins/healthstatelifeexpectanciesbyindexofmultipledeprivationimd/2018to2020#life-expectancy-at-birth-by-the-english-index-of-multiple-deprivation

ONS (2023) 'Childbearing for women born in different years, England

and Wales: 2023'. URL: ons.gov.uk/peoplepopulationandcommunity/birthsdeathsandmarriages/conceptionandfertilityrates/bulletins/childbearingforwomenbornindifferentyearsenglandandwales/2023

ONS (2024a) 'How is the fertility rate changing in England and Wales?' URL: ons.gov.uk/peoplepopulationandcommunity/birthsdeathsandmarriages/conceptionandfertilityrates/articles/howisthefertilityratechanginginenglandandwales/2024-10-28

ONS (2024b) 'Suicides in England and Wales: 2023 Registrations'. URL: ons.gov.uk/peoplepopulationandcommunity/birthsdeathsandmarriages/deaths/bulletins/suicidesintheunitedkingdom/2023

ONS (2025a) 'National life tables – life expectancy in the UK: 2021 to 2023'. URL: ons.gov.uk/peoplepopulationandcommunity/birthsdeathsandmarriages/lifeexpectancies/bulletins/nationallifetablesunitedkingdom/2021to2023additionaldata

ONS (2025b) 'Domestic abuse victim characteristics, England and Wales: year ending March 2025'. Office for National Statistics, 26 November. URL: ons.gov.uk/peoplepopulationandcommunity/crimeandjustice/articles/domesticabusevictimcharacteristicsenglandandwales/yearendingmarch2025

ONS (2026a) 'Female employment rate (aged 16 to 64, seasonally adjusted)'. URL: ons.gov.uk/employmentandlabourmarket/peopleinwork/employmentandemployeetypes/timeseries/lf25/lms

ONS (2026b) 'Male employment rate (aged 16 to 64, seasonally adjusted)'. URL: ons.gov.uk/employmentandlabourmarket/peopleinwork/employmentandemployeetypes/timeseries/mgsv/lms

Panah, R M, Jarvi, K et al (2024) 'Vitamin B_{12} is associated with higher serum testosterone concentrations and improved androgenic profiles among men with infertility'. National Library of Medicine September 2024. URL: pubmed.ncbi.nlm.nih.gov/38936552

Panahi, R (2023) '"Disgraceful front page" calls for "toxic masculinity" school classes'. Sky News Australia 5 September. URL: youtube.com/watch?v=HPNgpA4v72g

Pasquini, G & Kikuchi, E (2024) 'Who do Americans feel comfortable talking to about their mental health?' Pew Research Center 2 May. URL: pewresearch.org/short-reads/2024/05/02/who-do-americans-feel-comfortable-talking-to-about-their-mental-health/

Perheentupa, A, Mäkinen, J et al (2013) 'A cohort effect on serum testosterone levels in Finnish men'. National Library of Medicine 17 January. URL: pubmed.ncbi.nlm.nih.gov/23161753/

Ramírez-Soto, M C, Ortega-Cáceres, G & Arroyo-Hernández, H (2021) 'Sex differences in COVID-19 fatality rate and risk of death: An analysis in 73 countries, 2020–2021'. URL: pmc.ncbi.nlm.nih.gov/articles/PMC8805484

Rampell, C (2025) 'Why Gen Z men love Trump's reign of destruction'. *The Washington Post* 21 February. URL: washingtonpost.com/opinions/2025/02/21/trump-young-men-gen-z

Reeves, R V & Secker, W (2024) 'Male suicide: Patterns and recent trends'. American Institute for Boys and Men. URL: aibm.org/research/male-suicide.

Rezanezhad, B, Borgquist, R & Elzanaty, S (2023) 'Testosterone level and risk of diabetes: Follow-up study'. European Society of Medicine 28 September. URL: esmed.org/MRA/mra/article/view/4473

Rise Men's Health (2025) 'The role of stress in reducing testosterone levels and how to combat it'. 15 January. URL: risemenshealth.com/stress-in-reducing-testosterone-levels/

Roan, D (2025) '"Troubling decline" in secondary school PE lessons' *BBC* 8 June. URL: bbc.co.uk/sport/articles/cz634pyz51po

Samaritans (2025) 'Latest suicide data'. URL: samaritans.org/about-samaritans/research-policy/suicide-facts-and-figures/latest-suicide-data

Saxbe, D E, Edelstein R S et al (2017) 'Fathers' decline in testosterone and synchrony with partner testosterone during pregnancy predicts greater postpartum relationship investment'. National Library of Medicine April. URL: pubmed.ncbi.nlm.nih.gov/27469070

Schneider, M (2017) 'Google spent 2 years studying 180 teams. The most successful ones shared these 5 traits' *Inc* 19 July. URL: inc.com/michael-schneider/google-thought-they-knew-how-to-create-the-perfect.html

Schraer, R, Hix, C & Harris, L (2023) 'Antidepressants: Two million taking them for five years or more'. *BBC News* 19 June. URL: bbc.co.uk/news/uk-65825012

Scinicariello, F & Buser, M C (2016) 'Serum testosterone concentrations and urinary bisphenol A, benzophenone-3, triclosan, and paraben levels in male and female children and adolescents'. Environmental Health Perspectives Publishing 6 July. URL: ehp.niehs.nih.gov/doi/10.1289/EHP150

Secker, W & Williams, A (2024) 'Where are the men? Male representation in social work and psychology'. American Institute for Boys and Men January. URL: aibm.org/research/men-in-social-work-psychology

Shelter (2021) 'Women are some of the biggest losers in England's broken housing system'. 28 December. URL: england.shelter.org.uk/media/press_release/women_are_some_of_the_biggest_losers_in_englands_broken_housing_system

Shepherd, T (2025) 'One in three Australian men say they have committed intimate partner abuse, world-first research finds'. *The Guardian* 2 June. URL: theguardian.com/society/2025/jun/03/one-in-three-australian-men-say-they-have-committed-intimate-partner-violence-world-first-research-finds

Shultz, D (2016) 'Divorce rates double when people start watching porn, but is porn to blame for rocky marriages, or is it merely a symptom?' *Science Adviser* 26 August. URL: science.org/content/article/divorce-rates-double-when-people-start-watching-porn

Smailes, H & McGowan, M (2024) 'Strangulation during consensual sex in the UK: A report on findings from a pilot survey conducted in October 2024'. Institute for Addressing Strangulation. URL: ifas.org.uk/wp-content/uploads/2025/03/Strangulation-During-Sex-in-the-UK-December-2024-4-1.pdf

Starling Bank (2024) 'Gen Z men feel pressure to provide: 7 in 10 think "the man should be the breadwinner" in a family'. 19 February. URL: starlingbank.com/news/gen-z-men-feel-pressure-to-be-primary-providers-in-relationships

Statista Research Department (2025) 'Number of people reported to be sleeping rough in London from 2013/14 to 2024/25, by gender'. Statista, 10 September. URL: statista.com/statistics/381373/london-homelessness-rough-sleepers-by-gender

Strain, T, Flaxman, S et al (2024) 'National, regional, and global trends in insufficient physical activity among adults from 2000 to 2022: a pooled analysis of 507 population-based surveys with 5·7 million participants'. *The Lancet* Global Health August. URL: thelancet.com/journals/langlo/article/PIIS2214-109X%2824%2900150-5/fulltext

Susman, E (1995) 'Testosterone rises, falls with team'. UPI Archives 12 August. URL: upi.com/Archives/1995/08/12/Testosterone-rises-falls-with-team/1692808200000

Syed, M (2019) *Rebel Ideas*. John Murray.

Tannen, D (1990) *You Just Don't Understand*. Ballantine Books.

Thatcher, N (2025) 'Analysis: Pub numbers down by over 15,000 in past 25 years'. *The Morning Advertiser* 27 May. URL: morningadvertiser.co.uk/Article/2025/05/27/number-of-pub-closures-over-past-25-years

Thorn (2025) 'Sexual extortion & young people: Navigating threats in digital environments'. 24 June. URL: thorn.org/research/library/sexual-extortion-young-people

Ueda, P, Mercer, C H & C Ghaznavi, C (2020). 'Trends in frequency of sexual activity and number of sexual partners among adults aged 18 to 44 Years in the US, 2000-2018'. JAMA Network Open 3(6). URL: jamanetwork.com/journals/jamanetworkopen/fullarticle/2767066

UK Parliament (2012) 'Have kids, settle down: Marital and maternal age since 1938'. URL: parliament.uk/business/publications/research/olympic-britain/population/have-kids-settle-down

UNISON (2024) 'Closure of more than a thousand youth centres could have lasting impact on society' 15 June. URL: unison.org.uk/news/2024/06/closure-of-more-than-a-thousand-youth-centres-could-have-lasting-impact-on-society

Vasa, R A, Pine, D S et al (2011) 'Enhanced right amygdala activity in adolescents during encoding of positively valenced pictures'. *Developmental Cognitive Neuroscience* 1(1). URL: sciencedirect.com/science/article/pii/S1878929310000101

Venture Zero (2023) 'How to support Mental Health First Aiders in the workplace'. 5 April. URL: venturezero.co.uk/post/supporting-mental-health-first-aiders-in-the-workplace

Vinter, R (2026) 'Therapists who work with addiction report rise in out-of-control porn use by men'. *The Guardian* 3 January. URL: theguardian.com/society/2026/jan/03/more-than-half-of-uk-therapists-report-rise-in-out-of-control-porn-use

Vogels E A & McClain C (2023) 'Key findings about online dating in the U.S.' Pew Research Center 2 February. URL: pewresearch.org/short-reads/2023/02/02/key-findings-about-online-dating-in-the-u-s

Wahlstrom, D, Collins, P, White, T & Luciana, M (2011) 'Developmental Changes in Dopamine Neurotransmission in Adolescence: Behavioral Implications and Issues in Assessment'. National Library of Medicine 1 February. URL: pmc.ncbi.nlm.nih.gov/articles/PMC2815132

Walsh, S (2025) 'New study finds household plastics linked to heart disease deaths worldwide'. UPI Health News 29 April. URL: upi.com/Health_News/2025/04/29/plastics-study-heart-disease-deaths/9341745978421/

Walther, A, Breidenstein, J & Miller, R (2019) 'Association of Testosterone Treatment With Alleviation of Depressive Symptoms in Men: A Systematic Review and Meta-analysis'. *JAMA Psychiatry* Vol 76 No 1. January.

Weale, S (2023) 'Fathers have "unique effect" on children's educational outcomes, study finds'. *The Guardian* 20 September. URL: theguardian.com/society/2023/sep/20/fathers-have-unique-effect-on-childrens-educational-outcomes-study-finds

Weiss, G (2022) 'The Liver King, an influencer who eats raw meat and preaches a primal lifestyle, admits to lying about steroid use'. Business Insider 2 December. URL: businessinsider.com/influencer-the-liver-king-raw-diet-admits-steroid-use-2022-12

Weiss, R B (2021) 'Porn-induced erectile dysfunction: Can pornography impact male sexual performance?' *Psychology Today* 26 April. URL: psychologytoday.com/us/blog/love-and-sex-in-the-digital-age/202104/porn-induced-erectile-dysfunction

Whittaker, J, Costello, W & Thomas, A G (2024) 'Rethinking extremism: Predicting harm among incels (involuntary celibates): The roles of mental health, ideological belief and social networking. Commission for Countering Extremism. URL: assets.publishing.service.gov.uk/media/664e145fae748c43d37940af/140224%2BSISNET%2BIncel%2BReport.pdf

Whooten, R C, Kotelchuck, M et al (2023) 'Expectant fathers' health behaviors, infant care intentions, and social-emotional wellbeing in the perinatal period: A latent class analysis and comparison to mothers'. National Library of Medicine 26 August. URL: pmc.ncbi.nlm.nih.gov/articles/PMC10500477

Will, M (2023) 'Misogynist influencer Andrew Tate has captured boys' attention. What teachers need to know'. Education Week 2 February. URL: edweek.org/leadership/misogynist-influencer-andrew-tate-has-captured-boys-attention-what-teachers-need-to-know/2023/02

Wilson, M J & Scott, A J et al (2025) 'Suicidality in men following relationship breakdown: A systematic review and meta-analysis of global data'. *Psychological Bulletin* 151(7) URL: psycnet.apa.org/fulltext/2026-40673-001.html

Wood, L (2025) 'Abertay University research shows family movies stereotype males as predators and females as vulnerable prey'. Abertay University 6 June. URL: abertay.ac.uk/news/2025/abertay-university-research-shows-family-movies-stereotype-males-as-predators-and-females-as-vulnerable-prey

Work in Mind (2023) 'Nuffield Health's 2023 Healthier Nation Index: Only 36% of employees get a good night's sleep'. URL: workinmind.org/2023/09/08/nuffield-healths-2023-healthier-nation-index-only-36-of-employees-get-a-good-nights-sleep

World Health Organization (2024) 'Alcohol'. 28 June. URL: who.int/news-room/fact-sheets/detail/alcohol

Wright, M R & Hammersmith, A M et al (2019) 'The roles of marital dissolution and subsequent repartnering on loneliness in later life'. *The Journals of Gerontology Series B: Psychological Sciences and Social Sciences* 75(8). URL: pmc.ncbi.nlm.nih.gov/articles/PMC7489102/

Xu, X, Zhang, X et al (2018) 'Dynamic Patterns of Testosterone Levels in Individuals and Risk of Prostate Cancer among Hypogonadal Men: A Longitudinal Study'. *The Journal of Urology* 199(2). URL: pubmed.ncbi.nlm.nih.gov/28941925/

Yan, B W, Arias, E et al (2023) 'Widening gender gap in life expectancy in the US, 2010-2021'. Jama Internal Medicine 13 November. URL: jamanetwork.com/journals/jamainternalmedicine/fullarticle/2811338

Zečević, N, Veselinović, A et al (2025) 'Association Between zinc levels and the impact of its deficiency on idiopathic male infertility: An up-to-date review'. Multidisciplinary Digital Publishing Institute 29 January. URL: mdpi.com/2076-3921/14/2/165